Our Stem of Hope

The Andrew Curtis Story

Linda Curtis

About the author

Linda Curtis lived the dream until widowed in 2008 as a result of Motor Neurone Disease. Having re-evaluated life, perspectives and formulated new future plans, she now lives in Rockhampton with her two teenage children, toy poodles and cat and works in the education sector.

Published in Australia by Sid Harta Publishers Pty Ltd,
ABN: 46 119 415 842
23 Stirling Crescent, Glen Waverley, Victoria 3150 Australia
Telephone: +61 3 9560 9920, Facsimile: +61 3 9545 1742
E-mail: author@sidharta.com.au

First published in Australia 2017
This edition published 2017

Cover design, typesetting: WorkingType (www.workingtype.com.au)
Printed by Opus Group, Australia

Curtis, Linda
Our Stem of Hope — The Andrew Curtis Story
ISBN: 978-1-921030-69-7
pp196

Acknowledgements

Enormous thanks to Kerry Collison at Sid Harta Publishers, Barbara Ivusic and Luke Harris for their assistance in shining a light on Andrew's experience and allowing me to share our story with others. Thanks must also go to my family and friends for their unwavering support and love, during good times and bad and lastly, to Andrew, without whom there would have been no story to tell.

Dedication

To Hudson and Lainy;
Your dad was a truly special human being

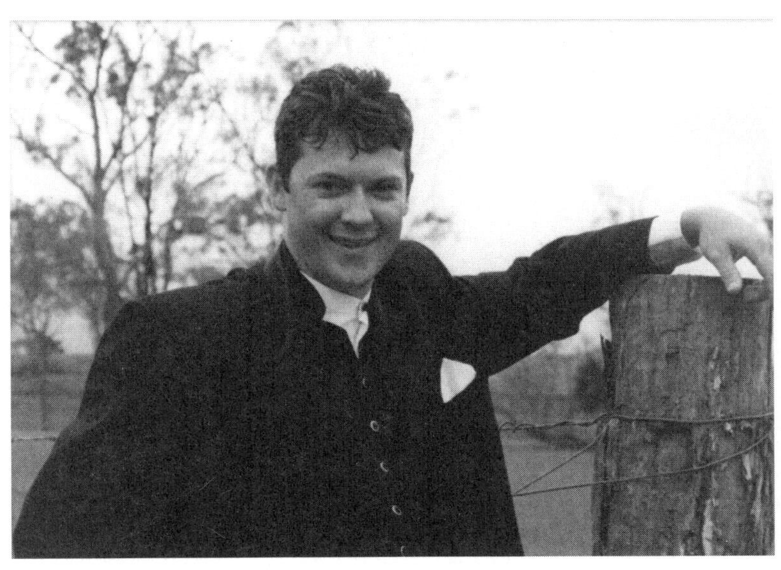

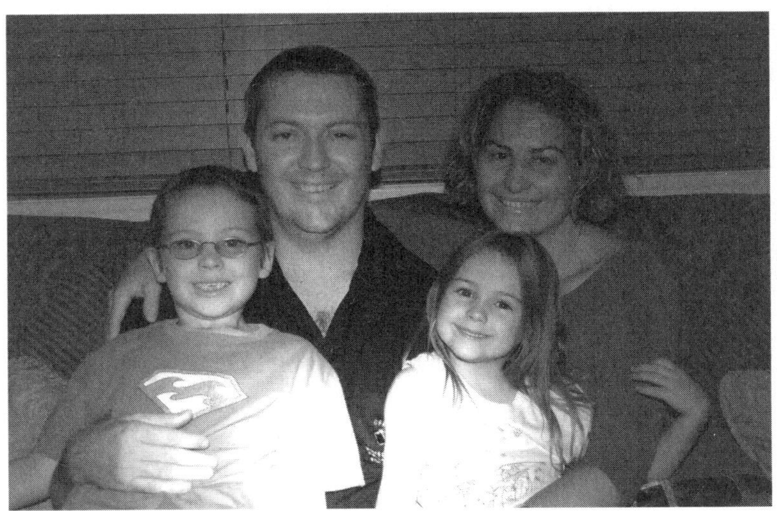

Contents

Introductions All Round 3
Children's Innocence, Lost 9
What's Going On? 13
Preliminary Assessments — M.N. What? 19
Hell Week — M.N.D., It Is 27
Change is Afoot 35
India, Take One 47
Home Again 55
Always Waiting 75
What Now? 83
India, Take Two 107
Home Once More 137
Permission Granted 157
'000' week 163
Running Out of Time 175

Prologue

Our room was full of people, but as we savoured your presence, we each could have been alone with you in an empty space. The atmosphere was palpable and the mood sombre, but most of us were oblivious to our surroundings as our individual memories, hopes, thoughts and emotions took precedence.

Just as we knew that you would never give up, we also knew that you could no longer go on. With much deliberation, this premise, along with a fathomless well of love, saw your mask removed for the very last time. After having tried so hard for so long to keep your mask on and knowing what its absence personified, seeing you without it was quite surreal and painful beyond words.

In that moment, you were both set free and condemned.

As you lay before me, I looked at you without the mask that had somehow become a part of you and I saw the man that you had always been — my partner in life and love, the father of my children and my hero. Acute sadness engulfed me as images of what should have been our future flashed before me — celebrating birthdays, anniversaries, attending graduations, teaching Hudson to shave, driving lessons, buying Hudson his first car, walking Lainy down the aisle at her wedding and just growing old and being together. At the same time, I was thankful for the life that we had shared and the many joys that we had experienced together. I was grateful that we had found one another so early on in our lives and the knowledge that what we had shared was very precious and rare was of great comfort. I was also overwhelmed with love and pride and I was in awe of your supreme strength of will, determination and non-defeatist attitude.

As I held your hand in mine and rested my other hand over your heart, time was suspended. You looked so peaceful; as though you were sleeping. But you weren't sleeping. With every beat of your heart and with every tear that fell, your life force was ebbing away.

Baboom… Baboom... Baboom... Baboom... and then you were gone.

Friday, 21st of November 2008, 7pm.

Introductions All Round

Prior to delving in and telling Andrew's story, I feel it's important to introduce him and give some insight into the type of person that he was and the person that he aspired to be. Firstly, however, I will present the family unit encompassing Andrew, as this was very much a part of who he was.

Hudson and Lainy — Our children

Hudson was born on the 9th of October, 2001. He has a sensitive nature, in that he internalises things and is aware of (and most times, is mindful of) others. Hudson tends to be a deep thinker and is quite accommodating in his attitudes.

Lainy was born on 6th of June, 2003 and is the spitting image of her dad. I often say that the only thing that she received from me was her belly button because she is 'Andrew in a dress'. She has quite a strong personality and is full of character, zeal and passion.

Merle and Roy — Andrew's parents

Together since Merle was thirteen and Roy was seventeen, they were married in 1958 and made their home in Mount Morgan. Their union produced eight children; Helen, Kenneth, Narelle, Suzanne, Gail, Allison, Gavin and Andrew. Funnily enough, they had only planned to have seven children.

The logistics involved in caring for a family of ten are difficult to comprehend and it was necessary for Merle and Roy to work as a team. Merle was responsible for domestic duties and she was the primary care-giver to the children while Roy worked hard to provide for his family. At one time, Roy was working three jobs at once!

When the Gold Mine closed down in Mount Morgan, Roy took a position at a Coal Mine in Blackwater in 1985. This was an enormous decision as it meant that the core family unit would be separated for the first time. Furthermore, due to Andrew's young age, it was determined that he too would relocate to Blackwater, despite resistance from Andrew and his siblings. Needless to say, he was not thrilled by the prospect of being separated from his siblings, but he did eventually settle in the new environment and after a time, made the most out of opportunities that were afforded him. The move also allowed Andrew to experience life as an only child — very different to the dynamics of being the eighth!

Merle has devoted her life to rearing her children and she continues the tradition by sharing her time and wisdom with her grandchildren and great-grandchildren. Roy has since retired and they moved back to Mount Morgan. He often wonders how he found time to go to work. He too imparts his wisdom and has the most fascinating tales to tell and a great repertoire of ditties.

Helen

Helen resides in Mount Morgan and has three adult children. She is a social worker employed in the health system. At the time of Andrew's illness, Helen and her sister, Narelle, were joint lease holders of the Golden Nugget Hotel in Mount Morgan.

Kenny (Kenneth)

Kenny is also a resident of Mount Morgan. Not unlike Andrew, one could say that he dances to the beat of his own drum.

Rel (Narelle)

Rel lives and works in Mount Morgan as a clinical nurse. She also has three adult children and for all intents and purposes, she appears to be the 'go to' person within the family.

Sue (Suzanne)

Sue resides in Biloela with her husband and is employed as a clinical nurse. She has two adult children.

Fan (Gail)

Fan resides in Gracemere with her husband and has three adult children.

Al (Allison)

Al lives in Gracemere with her son, but works in Mount Morgan as a nurse.

Gav (Gavin)

Gavin is also a Mount Morgan resident and like his brother, Andrew, found and married a 'nice Blackwater girl'. They have three children and while Gav is now employed in a different field, at the time of Andrew's illness, he was nursing.

Bill and Kath — My parents

Having lived and worked in the coalfields for the majority of their working life, one could say that dad was forcibly retired as a result of injuries sustained from a fall in 2005. They now reside in Rockhampton.

Tan (Tanya) — My sister

Tan resides in Tannum Sands, has three children and works in Gladstone.

Other relatives

In addition to our nuclear families, we are fortunate to have and maintain close relationships with many of our extended family members — they are not just misshapen branches on our family tree. Distance-wise, some are very close, like our then neighbour, Aunty Dawn, while others live further away. Regardless of where they are, we are all connected and share a special bond.

In our case, the old adages, 'Family's stick together', 'Fight one, fight all' and 'Blood is thicker than water', all proved true. While our journey was not an easy one, having such unwavering support enabled us to make it through the darkest of days. At times, one would never had thought it possible that you could maintain vigilance or survive such events, but when things became unbearable, the scaffolding surrounding each of us as individuals allowed us to take a step back, regroup and join the front line again, once our energy sources were renewed. Someone always had your back.

It is difficult to explain, but once Andrew's plight was realised, the persons closest to him literally halted their own lives and the universal focus was on supporting Andrew. The level of commitment demonstrated by our family was staggering, especially when you consider that there were no time-frames — they were in it for the long haul. Andrew's wellbeing and comfort was our common goal and in order to achieve it, our home literally became the home of our family. My parents resided with us during the week and helped out with the kids and school. Andrew's parents visited every day and Merle took over the kitchen duties; making sure we were all well looked after in that department. Everyone contributed, giving as little or as much as they could. Work commitments were negotiated and schedules changed to enable sufficient (medical) coverage for Andrew and when people were 'rostered on' their families were also often present.

Given that Andrew's being hospitalised was not an option that we considered, our caring for him at home would not have been possible without the expertise and willingness of his siblings to provide the care he required, their boundless commitment and the understanding and support of spouses'/partners, children and the Mount Morgan and Biloela Hospitals.

Andrew

Capable; Loyal; Proud; Passionate; Honest; Strong; Determined; Intelligent; Bold; Opinionated; Iron-willed; Leader; Inspirational — but a few words, that for me, encapsulate the essence that is Andrew.

Andrew Richard Curtis was the youngest child of Merle and Roy and as such, was his parents and seven elder siblings "baby". He was most often endearingly referred to as "Bub", which was quite comical given that he was the biggest of all his siblings. He spent his primary school years in Mount Morgan and prior to starting secondary school, moved with his parents to Blackwater. Here he completed his formative schooling, attained an apprenticeship and became a Diesel Fitter. He toiled in this field at both underground and open cut coal mine sites around the Blackwater area.

Throughout his work life, Andrew was an active member of the Construction Forestry, Mining and Energy Union (C.F.M.E.U.) and an avid believer of their fundamental principles. He held various positions within the organisation and at the time of his illness, was in the role of President of the Blackwater Number 1 Lodge, as well as a host of other positions at a local, district and national level. The C.F.M.E.U. was an integral part of Andrew's life.

On a personal level, nothing was more important to Andrew than his family — nuclear, extended and those special few that he considered to be a part of his inner circle. We could have been the poster couple for 'high school sweethearts', having been together for over half of our lives. Who knew that our tryst on that Wednesday afternoon, twenty-plus years ago, would result in such a permanent pairing. Funnily enough, that afternoon was one of the only times I can recall 'wagging' school. Andrew absolutely adored and doted on our children, Hudson and Lainy. They were his proudest accomplishment and his greatest joy. Andrew also loved being 'at home' in Mount Morgan surrounded by his extended family and whenever the opportunity arose, we were there. There wasn't a thing that he wouldn't do for any of us.

Andrew was, and always had been, extremely adept at expressing his views and opinions and he relished a good argument (which I'm sure many would assent to). His recall ability was phenomenal and it served him well in both his personal and professional lives. It was also quite beneficial, albeit frustrating for others, when having said arguments and sitting down for a few hands of 500 (his favoured card game).

Passion was one of Andrew's fortes. He was passionate about things that he cared about and believed in — family, C.F.M.E.U., Fords, St George/ Illawara Dragons (football team) — and he always fought for what he thought was right and just, regardless of the consequences. Fortunately, he had a way with words and could pretty much talk his way out of anything and this attribute was his saviour on many occasions.

Love him or not, the way Andrew conducted himself and his achievements garnered the respect of many. The combination of traits that he possessed, his delivery and the way he handled himself was the bane of some persons' existence, but by the same token, his idiosyncrasies and tenacity enabled him to assist countless others and make a real difference in people's lives. He was a truly gifted and special individual and the behaviour, courage and spirit he exhibited throughout his illness adds testament to this.

Children's Innocence, Lost

"My Daddy's a legend!"

Whether it was playing cricket or soccer in the backyard, teaching the finer art of bike riding, answering obscure questions about everything and anything, telling stories or battling on the PS2 (all fundamental attributes in the eyes of a child), the aforementioned catch cry would reign. According to our children, there was nothing Andrew didn't know and there was nothing that he couldn't do (and yes, this could be quite exasperating at times!). While this continues to be the case and the pedestal that their Dad is on remains intact, Andrew's illness rocked our children's world to its foundations.

All that you wish for as a parent is safe passage for your child; in every sense. Your aim is to nurture them and provide them with everything (and more) that they need to grow and blossom through each milestone. To facilitate their meandering through each transitional phase, you try to teach them about life and protect them from unnecessary hurt and anguish. Yes, the latter are a part of life and yes, children need to experience them in order to develop mechanisms to cope with them, but when your child is confronted with the mortality of one of their creators, how can you shield them from that? How can you explain it, when you don't understand it yourself?

Innocence is synonymous with childhood, but sadly, the innocence of our children has been lost as they are forced to confront issues that we as adults can barely compute.

People often say that children are resilient and they will

adapt, and through my experience, I have found this to be true to a certain extent. However, such a blanket statement in some ways minimises their ordeal. It doesn't acknowledge the pain and confusion they endure, or the uncertainty they face, or recognise the things that they have each had to develop to overcome or exist with such a harsh reality. It also negates to take into account the high level of support bestowed on them in an effort to provide them with some sense of security, stability and normality.

We decided early on not to keep Andrew's illness from Hudson and Lainy as we felt they needed to know what was happening. It was obvious that there was something amiss and it didn't take long for the kids to notice and make comments regarding their observations. We didn't inundate them with the intricate details, but we provided them with information on a level that they could understand. We also made sure they were exposed to the reality of Andrew's illness, although this was closely monitored. Throughout the course of his illness, the kids became actively involved in some aspects of Andrew's care.

We tried to be as honest as possible with the kids as we didn't want to trivialise what was happening or provide them with false hope. This was a struggle as the need to protect them was sometimes overwhelming. When Lainy asked, "What if Daddy doesn't get better?", we would have liked nothing better than to say, "Of course he'll get better. Daddy's not going anywhere." However, such a reassurance wouldn't have been fair or truthful. Instead, we tried to explain that it wasn't Daddy's choice to be unwell and he was trying everything he could to get better, but we didn't know if the special medicine would be able to help him. We continually reinforced Andrew's love for the kids and his desire to get well so he could share in the experience of their lives.

In the face of everything, I am thankful that Hudson and Lainy are secure in the knowledge that their dad loved them more than anything and he would have given the world to stay with us. Once, when asked about their Dad, Hudson said that Andrew loved them and would never have left us if he had had the choice. This revelation comforts me to no end as it signifies that the kids are safe in the knowledge that their Dad loved them more than life itself.

Andrew's illness has impacted heavily on all of us, but none more so than the children. Not just Hudson and Lainy, but all of Andrew's nieces and nephews, irrespective of age. Most visited when they could and Tay (Rel's daughter) especially would spend hours on end just being in the room with Andrew. We dubbed Lilah (Gav's daughter) 'Matron Sloan' as she would march into Andrew's room as soon as they arrived and would insist on being put on his bed. She took pride of place beside him on his pillow and she would chatter to him, kiss his mask, rub his arms, play with him and watch TV. They loved the cooking channels, which was ironic as Andrew was unable to indulge.

Lilah was only around twenty months old, but she was very protective of Andrew and would rouse on others for getting on the bed, or on the adults for doing things to him, even when it was for his own good. Theirs was a very special bond and the connection continued after Andrew's passing. During a visit, a few days afterwards, we couldn't find Lilah anywhere in the house. We found her out in the shed, sitting in the middle of Andrew's bed (which has since been donated to the Palliative Care Ward at the Mt Morgan Hospital). Similarly, Sienna (Lilah's sister) walked past our closed bedroom door and made the comment that something was very different now.

Kids are amazing, intuitive and precious creatures and while we cannot always save them from trauma and tragedy, we can walk beside them, share the experience, be understanding, guide and support them. Oftentimes, however, I wonder who supports whom?

What's Going On?

For the latter part of 2007, Andrew had been extremely busy with his union work and it wasn't uncommon for him to be travelling here, there and everywhere in performing his duties. Among other things, he was one of the team members negotiating the Enterprise Bargaining Agreement for BMA and this took up an enormous amount of his time. Although he was a diesel fitter, I often joked that I'd have to go and label his tools and he'd have to do a refresher course as he'd not had cause to use them for a long time due to his union commitments. Essentially, the spanners were replaced by the tools of his new trade — his mind and his mouth.

It's hard to say when Andrew's symptoms first presented themselves or exactly what the initial warning signs were. Due to his workload and the heightened stress associated with it, anything that may have been happening early on was likely attributed to this. Andrew being afflicted by something sinister never entered our minds. Rather, we ventured a guess that he may have some obscure fatigue issue that was being exacerbated by the stress he was experiencing. I recall many conversations whereby I encouraged (or as he would say, "nagged") him to go and see a doctor regarding his complaints, but he was always much too busy.

November 2007

Andrew was hospitalised for three days with a roaring temperature that couldn't be broken and was accompanied by a rash. Innumerable tests were performed; to no avail. For want of a better verdict, we were advised that Andrew had tonsillitis and was allergic to penicillin, but we weren't convinced that this was an accurate diagnosis. I guess we'll never know the true cause of Andrew's illness or what bearing this episode had or didn't have on his future health.

Due to the nature of his work, Andrew spent a good deal of time taking and making phone calls (this is a slight understatement as the phone was his faithful companion — the Bat Phone). It was during one such call that brought our attention to his slurring speech. Mid way through the conversation, the person asked Andrew if he had been drinking as he was slurring his words. He assured them that he hadn't been, but the fact remained that his speech was affected. We hadn't picked up on this ourselves, but once it was brought to our attention, it was obvious. We noted that the slurring emerged and became more prominent whenever Andrew was upset or tired, but it was not constant.

Mid December 2007

This is when one of the first physical signs was noticed. Andrew was in Brisbane on Union business and his sister, Rel, her girls and I joined him there for a few days of shopping. During a trip out, Rel happened to be walking behind Andrew and she noticed that he was walking differently; his gait had changed and he was flicking out his right foot. Also, after walking only a short distance, it was necessary for us to stop so that Andrew could rest. He literally could not walk as he was too tired. He was short of breath, his body was shaking, he was sweating profusely and he had a feeling of extreme weakness in his extremities. We returned to our apartment so Andrew could rest and while his condition improved, he didn't venture out again. This was very unlike him, especially when one of our jaunts was to be a visit to the casino.

Late December 2007

Andrew didn't dwell on the Brisbane episode and throughout the remainder of the month, he carried on as he always did; work, meetings, travel, meetings, meetings, travel, work. However, his schedule was intermittently disrupted by periods of debilitating fatigue. On occasion, the mundane action of walking up the stairs became a herculean effort. As we lived in a high house, it was sometimes necessary for Andrew to pull himself upwards by the railings and go one step at a time. Upon reaching the top, he would have to go and lay down for a few hours to recuperate, as he could not physically function without rest. It was so unlike him to be unwell and while he was concerned, he was also very frustrated as his condition was beginning to have a negative impact and his being unable to put a name to what was happening was further cause for aggravation.

Following one of his many trips to Brisbane, Andrew voiced his concern that he may be having a relapse of glandular fever. He first suffered from this affliction several years ago, and had had recurring bouts previously.

Andrew's lethargy was also noted during the Christmas period and he was happier to stay on the sidelines than join in with the usual Christmas activities, which was quite out of character. It was around this time also that we noticed changes in Andrew's posture; his shoulders were rounded as opposed to square.

New Year's Eve 2007

In what would appear to be a direct contradiction to everything else that Andrew was experiencing, on New Year's Eve, we took the kids on an adventure to the Blackdown Tablelands and hiked to Rainbow Falls — over 4km round trip. Andrew ended up carrying our little princess half the distance, as she couldn't possibly walk all that way on her own! Surprisingly, apart from a general lack of fitness (which we were both guilty of), Andrew showed no overt signs of distress from the trek.

Late January 2008

Andrew was in Brisbane on Union business and following a short walk from the office to his apartment, he experienced jelly legs and extreme fatigue (as though he had just run a gruelling marathon), breathing difficulty and he had trouble turning the key in the lock to his room. He contacted Rel in the midst of the episode, relaying what was happening and advising that he had no strength in his right hand and that things were just 'not right'. Andrew returned to Rockhampton, but due to work commitments he had to depart for Blackwater almost immediately, thus not allowing any tests or medical follow up to be conducted. Regarding the call, Rel remembers alarm bells starting to ring as she collated the information and added it to the rapidly expanding list of unexplained things that Andrew had already experienced.

On returning to Rockhampton for a personal visit a few days later, Andrew experienced another episode whereby he was virtually rendered immobile from fatigue following a very brief period of physical exertion. Plans were made and Andrew went to hospital and underwent a barrage of tests — all of which came back negative. At the time, we were very concerned and bewildered by what was occurring as there continued to be no plausible explanation for it.

Andrew continued to feel 'out of sorts', but he soldiered on, going to work and attending meetings. He met the kids and I at their school for their first day — Hudson in Grade One and Lainy in Prep. On arrival, he had to walk a short distance to meet up with us and by the time he did, he was very pale, sweaty and nauseous. It must have been quite obvious that there was something wrong as more than one person commented on his condition. I recall taking photos of Andrew with the kids — sitting at Hudson's desk and helping Lainy fill her water bottle — and his not being too happy about it. I'm glad I insisted.

Andrew feeling poorly didn't stop him from meeting previous obligations as he travelled to and from Bundaberg the following day to attend to business.

Preliminary Assessments – M. N. What?

Amidst the excitement of Hudson losing his first tooth, Andrew's health continued to decline. In addition to his fatigue (that seemed to be a constant companion), he was experiencing muscle twitches, cramps and his slurred speech was occurring more regularly. Andrew finally gave in to demands and agreed to see a doctor about what was happening, on the provision it occur after his scheduled trip to Brisbane on the 7th of February 2008.

Saturday 9th of February

I had already been in to see a doctor with Lainy and mum had taken her and Hudson off shopping while we had Andrew's consultation. Obviously, we were not expecting anything out of the ordinary to come of it, or we would never have arranged dual appointments and had the children with us. Andrew and I waited in the doctor's surgery, watching people going in and coming out only a few minutes later. We weren't so lucky. Following our purge of information, the doctor requested Andrew poke out his tongue. To our astonishment, Andrew's tongue was seemingly alive as it moved and wriggled about; resembling a bag of worms. This was the first time we heard the word, 'fasciculation' and added to the fact that it was indicative of a neurological issue, we would rather have stayed ignorant. Things such as 'brain tumour', 'multiple sclerosis' and 'auto-immune disorder' were cited as possible causes for what Andrew was experiencing, but nothing could be confirmed without tests, which the doctor ordered — an MRI on Tuesday.

We left the surgery feeling quite literally shocked, numb and terrified. We were more unsure than ever about what was happening and the notion that it could be one of the things the doctor had suggested was preposterous. The sense of helplessness, even at this early stage was almost tangible as we knew something was terribly wrong, but we didn't know why or how or what and we couldn't find out because we had to wait for tests. Despite this and what he must have been feeling, Andrew was ever the protector as he tried to comfort and reassure me. It was all very surreal and in the midst of trying to process everything that had transpired, we had to face the kids too!

Still reeling (and somewhat dazed), we parted ways and did what we had previously planned for the morning — I went with mum and the kids and Andrew returned to Mum and Dad's. On our way home, Rel rang me and said that Andrew had called her in quite a distressed state, relaying the morning events and what the doctor had alluded to. Having been enshrined in my own haze since the consultation, Rel's call compounded my fear as it forced me to realise that Andrew was scared too. Somehow, knowing that he was so fearful alarmed me even more — because to me, Andrew was invincible. I recall sitting at the traffic lights on Yaamba Road, trying to keep it together for the sake of the kids, while telling Mum that things could be really, really bad because all indications were that Andrew had some type of neurological issue.

Meeting up with Andrew again when we arrived at Mum's was quite a poignant moment as we'd both had some time to digest things. We didn't say much to each other, but then we didn't have to. It's true that a look can communicate a thousand words. We were also very conscious that the kids were ever-present and we didn't want to frighten them by totally wigging out. I was grateful that Mum and Dad were there to entertain them, which gave Andrew and I some much-needed space.

We decided to go to the Mount and during the trip up there, I remember holding Andrew's hand and watching him and every now and again he'd catch my eye and we'd just gaze. I was amazed by how much more I was taking in — really looking at the little things that seem to get lost or go unnoticed every other day. Everything was so much more precious.

We opted to stay at Rel's instead of Andrew's parents for a few reasons. We didn't want to burden Merle and Roy with unnecessary worry and grief and as such, Andrew made the decision to not tell them of his visit to the Doctor until after the scheduled tests — he wanted to be able to give them as much information as he could. Andrew also felt comfortable there given his close bond with Rel and his health status.

As it was Georja's (Rel's youngest daughter) birthday the next day, there was a BBQ at Rel's that night. Everyone was there apart from Sue as she was working. It felt good to be surrounded by family and be a part of the normality, but it was quite a difficult night to get through as it was hard to keep the emotions in check.

Andrew had pondered and had decided to protect his parents from what was happening until he had something more concrete to tell them, but he had no such qualms in sharing with his siblings; The Unit. All of those present at the BBQ, gathered together (it was all a bit secret squirrel) in one of the bedrooms and we let them know what had transpired thus far. Like us, everyone was in disbelief, shocked and upset, but from the moment we informed them, their support was solid. While we knew that they would support us no matter what, it was comforting to have them all validate it, and vehemently so.

As one could imagine, we wanted to know everything

about everything regarding Andrew's circumstances and in not receiving anything from the medical fraternity at this juncture, we took it upon ourselves to do as much research and gain as much information as we could. We couldn't just sit idle and wait around. Knowledge is power and as we were in a very powerless position, we were hungry for it. We all spent a lot of time on the computer (Rel practically took up residence in the study) looking for everything and anything to do with Andrew's condition and symptoms. At one point, Andrew intimated that from his research, he knew what he had (meaning Motor Neurone Disease — M.N.D.). As strange as it may seem, we were hoping that the tests would show that Andrew had some form of brain tumour, as at least with this affliction, there was a chance it could be operable and to us it seemed like the lesser nasty.

The hours of pouring over information on the internet did nothing to allay our fears. In one sense, it was good to be doing something proactive, but on the other hand, little of the information provided us with much hope. At times, it was like the more you read, the more terrifying Andrew's predicament became. We told each other we shouldn't worry until we knew what we were facing and we need to wait to find out what the tests reveal and so on and so forth, but we were all doing exactly that. I wished many times to wake up from the nightmare, only to realise that it was all too real and our lives were forever changed, regardless of what any tests showed. Andrew was sick. He was really sick.

Sunday 10th of February; Georja's birthday

The night of Georja's birthday saw Andrew have oxygen for the first time. He became quite distressed as he felt as though he wasn't getting enough breath so we attended the hospital and he was provided oxygen. We're not exactly sure why it happened, what caused it or how big a role anxiety played (if any), but the treatment seemed to alleviate Andrew's breathlessness and he felt better afterwards.

Come Monday, given that we had waited nearly two days already, we tried to have the M.R.I. brought forward. We were all desperately afraid of what the M.R.I. would, or wouldn't show, and having to wait for another day for the test to be administered was excruciating. As it turned out, it couldn't be rescheduled due to logistics — I felt like screaming. Did they not realise how much we needed to know what was going on? Did they even care? It wasn't like we were waiting to see if Andrew's arm was broken! This was our life!

Tuesday 12th of February

Sue came up from Biloela and had the kids while we went to the hospital for the M.R.I. We had our own little posse as Rel came with us and Mum and Dad met us at the hospital. We were thankful for the support. The test seemed to take forever and once it had been completed, nobody could tell us anything and we were advised that the results wouldn't be available for a few days. We found this to be totally unacceptable. Again, did people not realise the significance of these test results for us? Were they so complacent that we were really only a number to them? Surely, they could sense our desperation and need? Apparently not, as this was the protocol.

Bollocks to that! We presented at the surgery that we had initially attended, but the doctor we had seen was absent. By chance, one of the Doctor's at the surgery was known to Rel and after telling him of our plight, he agreed to see us and contact the hospital in relation to Andrew's test results. They were negative. Thus, it appeared that whatever Andrew's affliction, it wasn't a brain tumour or multiple sclerosis.

After discussions, the doctor concurred that M.N.D. was at

the forefront as a possible diagnosis, but further tests would be necessary to establish this (while there is no definitive test for M.N.D., the diagnosis is basically made by ruling out all other possibilities).

Walking to the car after leaving the surgery, Andrew made the understatement of all time. He said that things were totally *#*#ed and that he was going to be "ripped off". He also made mention of the kids and how he had to be around to see them grow up. It was all very emotional, as it seemed that our worst fears were being realised and there was nothing we could do to stop it. Things were totally out of control and there didn't appear to be any way to rein it in. While we all tried to be brave for one another and support each other, we were all sick inside. I knew I was as the hollow sensation in my stomach had intensified a thousand-fold. I knew also that things were only going to get worse as we entered the next phase — the vast unknown.

Given what we now knew, we could no longer put off the inevitable. Merle and Roy needed to be told what was going on. But, Andrew was their baby. How could we tell them that he likely had a terminal illness? What would we tell them? Who would tell them? How would they react to the news? We considered our options and tried to find the least brutal way of letting them know what was happening. In the end, Rel went out and saw them and we followed a short time afterwards. It was an extremely arduous time for us all and one of the times I wish never to have to live through again. It was an enormously draining day and Andrew was very tired. We all were.

Not content to wait around and go through the process at a pace determined by 'the system', the next day, Rel enlisted the assistance of our local G.P. with the aim of getting Andrew to Brisbane to be assessed as soon as possible. So, while the kids frolicked in the flooded creek and kept busy with their cousins, we researched doctors and hospitals and established that the Royal Brisbane and Women's Hospital (R.B.H.) was best suited to our needs as their Neurological Department and staff were at the forefront with regard to M.N.D. research. We initiated contact and liaised directly with the hospital with the aim of expediting the referral process because as we saw it, we didn't have time to wait. We barely had the patience to wait a day, let alone a month!

In the interim, I returned to Blackwater to pack some more gear, pay some bills and generally bring things up to speed. During this time, I contacted my employer and advised that I was unable to present for work due to personal circumstances and I was unable to give a return date. Andrew also made contact with his employer and the Union, citing the same.

The atmosphere at Rel's was very intense and while we tried to shield the kids from the bulk of it, it was inevitable that they would pick up the vibe that things were far from okay. Just the fact that we were staying at Rel's and not Ma Merle's already had them suspicious. While we were open with the kids from the outset and they were very much aware that Daddy was unwell and we weren't sure of the reason, we didn't want them directly exposed to the constant and extreme levels of anxiety that we were all subject to. Thus, we decided it best for them to go and stay with my parents for a few days. As much as we wanted them close to us, we further decided that they should return home to Blackwater (with my parents) and attend school as they would benefit from the normality and stability of the routine that this offered.

Andrew had bouts of extreme tiredness throughout the day and had claimed one of the lounge chairs. He didn't venture far from it, apart from when we attended the hospital for more oxygen treatment. While our levels were nowhere near Andrew's, just waiting around for people to contact us was very anxiety-provoking and exhausting.

Thursday 14th of February

Valentine's Day arrived and for us, it assumed a very different connotation to that which it had had in previous years. We were much more mindful and attuned to one another and given all that was going on, we were closer than ever. Suddenly, receiving roses or a gift seemed ridiculous. The only thing that I wanted was for things to be the same as they were. Seemingly, something I couldn't have.

The R.B.H. contacted and advised that we could present that afternoon or tomorrow, but we couldn't be guaranteed a bed. Further negotiations ensued and it was determined that Andrew would be admitted through Accident and Emergency (A & E) the following Monday and flight and accommodation bookings were arranged. While it was good to know that we would soon be going to Brisbane and getting closer to finding out what the hell was going on, the incessant waiting was daunting and very taxing on everyone.

The days prior to our going to Brisbane were filled with family. Given that we didn't know what the future had in store for us, we decided early on that regardless of the outcome, we would try to make every day a good day and be thankful for what we had. I picked the kids up from my parents on the Friday and we all visited Merle and Roy's every day. Many of our relatives and friends from afar contacted via phone and a few made the trip to see us before we left.

Mum and Dad collected the kids on Sunday and took them to Blackwater. It was very difficult to let them go and there were more than a few hugs, kisses and tears. Everyone else congregated at Merle's that night for a get-together. The mood of the evening was quite odd as it wasn't a happy occasion by any means, but everyone was happy to be together. Andrew's health hadn't improved any, but despite this, he became involved in some of the festivities, even playing a few hands of 500.

Hell Week — M.N.D., It Is

Monday 18th of February

The day that Helen welcomed another grandchild, saw us arrive in Brisbane and begin one of the most harrowing and emotionally ravaging weeks of our lives. Andrew, Rel & I presented to the R.B.H. A & E Department around 3pm as per prior discussions regarding Andrew's admission to the Neurological Ward — 7B North. In doing so, we essentially bypassed the process of referral from GP to Specialist, as well as the associated waiting period, which was our main concern. Given our circumstances, waiting for weeks/months to see our choice of specialist was a luxury we couldn't afford.

Not surprisingly, we had to wait once we arrived at A & E. We were like cats on a hot tin roof, although a visit from some close friends helped us to pass the time and take our mind off things. Once Andrew was called, we were allocated a curtained space and after another short wait, were seen by the Specialist and two accompanying Doctors. The consult was very thorough and we tried to provide as much information as possible; physical and verbal. There was also a lot to take in as the Doctors' advised of and explained the tests that Andrew would be undergoing and likely time frames of them occurring. With regard to a diagnosis, they concurred that while Andrew certainly appeared to have symptoms of M.N.D., they could not yet say yes or no as to whether this was what he had. They further advised that a consult with another neurologist from the Princess Alexandra (P.A.) Hospital had been scheduled for later in the week.

Following the consultation, Andrew was admitted and we were settled into his room by 5pm — Bed 41. Andrew had requested a private room and we were very thankful that this came to fruition. It was difficult enough being in the hospital setting, knowing what traumatic tests awaited, not knowing whether what was happening was life or death, let alone having to experience this in a shared room with strangers. Although, I guess that anyone sharing a room (and a bathroom) in such circumstances wouldn't remain strangers for long. I remember walking to Andrew's room, feeling for everyone else that was on the ward, not knowing their stories and quite frankly, not really wanting to know. I knew how hard it was for us just at that moment and quite selfishly, wouldn't and couldn't take on any more.

Andrew was totally drained as it had been an enormous day and Rel and I were also on the other side of tired, but it was still extremely tough to leave him and retire to our motel. Neither of us wanted to leave him at the hospital alone and while Andrew said otherwise, we were sure he didn't want us to go. If we could have stayed with him in the hospital we would have because no matter what, I guess we had made an unconscious pledge to never leave Andrew alone. Never let him feel that he was alone. Like us, I'm sure he didn't get much sleep that night.

We rang Andrew first thing, just to see how he was travelling and to reiterate that we would be there as soon as visiting hours allowed (although, we didn't put too much stock in these hours as we figured we would be there whenever and for however long Andrew needed us to be). Gav also made the trek down today. The more the merrier. With each of us present, the load seemed to be just that much less. Personally, it was very comforting to have Rel and Gav with us because apart from the practical support, in a medical sense they were able to translate things, putting it in lei terms so that Andrew and I (more specifically, I) could understand what was happening. Let me say that feeling totally out of your depth and not being able to do anything about it is absolutely dismaying. Having their support alleviated these feelings somewhat, but that feeling of helplessness was relentless.

The first scheduled test that Andrew had was the 'muscle test'. It basically consisted of Andrew's muscles being shocked to elicit a response. Needle-like apparatus were inserted directly into his muscles and were then subject to electric impulses. As painful as the procedure must have been, Andrew pretty much grinned and bared it. I think I showed more emotion and I was just watching! The results of the test showed that Andrew had nerve damage on his right side. Given that this was the side that we had recognised the most weakness, this was not a surprise, but having it verified was unsettling and added to our fears.

I guess people deal with fear and adversity in varying ways and as horrifying as our situation appeared to be, we seemed to fall back on humour as a way of helping us through. Thus, in the hostile hospital environment, we reverted to ways of comfort. We played cards (as only Curtis' could), told stories and basically joked around to counteract the demoralising reality. Staff must have thought it strange hearing guffawing laughter within the realms of ward 7B North. To us though, it gave us a reprieve.

Thursday 21st of February

Andrew had no scheduled tests Wednesday, but Thursday saw him have a lumbar puncture — or eight! Over the course of Thursday, various doctors came in with the aim of performing a lumbar puncture (to test his spinal fluid for adverse elements). The procedure was difficult and intensely painful, but eight times, PLEASE! The most surprising thing though, for me, was Andrew's response, or lack thereof and his accommodation of the procedure happening more than three, let alone eight times!

He was surprising me at every turn. Just when I thought I knew what to expect, and was waiting for the explosion, it didn't come. Instead, Andrew demonstrated a level of patience that I didn't think he possessed. Once the test was completed successfully, results showed his spinal fluid to be clear, which further alluded to M.N.D.

Thursday was also our "D-Day", with regard to the neurologist from the P.A. coming to consult on Andrew's case. Notwithstanding the respect that she rightfully deserves, we dubbed her role in our non-fiction actuality as that of "Doctor Death". She earned this title as she basically corroborated the diagnosis of M.N.D.

Actual confirmation that Andrew had M.N.D. was shocking. It was like all the air had been sucked out of the room and even though the doctors kept talking, things were silent and all I could hear was M.N.D., M.N.D., M.N.D., M.N.D. echoing. I shudder to think what it must have been like for Andrew. While things had been highly suggestive of this diagnosis, I don't know that there is any way to really prepare yourself for such news. Up until the very last second, I was hoping that everyone would realise that there had been some huge mistake and that while Andrew wasn't fine, he certainly didn't have a terminal illness. The realisation that M.N.D. and all that it entailed was now inescapable was truly devastating.

Once the doctors left and Rel and Gav stepped out to give us some space, Andrew and I pretty much fell apart. We just lay on the bed holding each other and crying. Our main concern was the kids and the unfairness of Andrew not having the time to watch them grow up. Knowing that Hudson and Lainy would not have the opportunity to experience their Dad personally as they grew older was desperately painful. This, and the fact that Andrew was also going to miss out on his 'babies' future lives was the most difficult to bare.

While trying to understand that Andrew had essentially been put on the 'short list' and what that meant for him and us and our family, I was also besieged by selfish thoughts like: How can I live without him? How can I cope without him? We've been a team for so long, what will I do without him beside me? He's my back up. He's my rock. This is Andrew we're talking about — how can he not beat this? I never thought I would be alone. I never thought I would have to do it all by myself. I can't do it by myself. Selfish. Selfish. Selfish. This was torturous and of course, I kept these thoughts to myself, but I've no doubt that every question I asked myself crossed Andrew's mind as well. What must he have been thinking? I don't know if I want to know.

Andrew didn't dwell, as was his nature. Remarkably, within hours of his diagnosis, he was brainstorming and making plans and looking for ways to fight. Even though the doctors had intimated at what lay ahead, Andrew wasn't willing to just take that on board, sit back and wait for things to happen. His intrinsic fighting spirit was shining through.

From all accounts, M.N.D. is quite an individual disease in the sense that each person may experience different symptoms in varying degrees at different stages. You could have ten people with the disease, but they may all display different symptoms or be affected by each symptom in their own way. It's almost as though it is personalised as no two cases are exactly the same. Thus, we didn't know what to expect or when to expect it, which made things even more difficult to comprehend because we didn't know what exactly we were up against. Contrary to this, the idiosyncratic nature of the disease also gave us hope. The future was basically unwritten, as we couldn't really compare Andrew's case with other sufferers of the disease.

Friday saw Andrew take a breathing test, see an Occupational and Speech Therapist and start medication that may, or may not help his condition, but given it was the only thing on offer, we decided 'what the hell'. He was also released from the hospital and I remember Rel having words with the resident pharmacist regarding the provision of Andrew's medication because as usual, there was a drama! Despite the enormity of the day, at Andrew's insistence we dined out at one of his favourite restaurants — Brekky Creek Wharf — we were joined by extended family and close friends. While things were totally removed from normality with regard to our situation, it was nice to sit and talk and be involved in something that was familiar to us, in that we had done the same thing many times in the past.

The realisation that our lives were changing and many of the contributing elements were unknown was one we acknowledged early on (even though sometimes we chose not to see it, as it was just easier). To counter this, we started to talk about and make plans for things that we could control. Thus, our time in Brisbane wasn't just spent waiting around and going from one medical appointment or procedure to the next. We needed to be practical and realistic, which meant discussing life issues such as our employment, where we would live and the kids' schooling.

We found the internet to be an invaluable tool as we scouted real estate in 'God's Country' (Mount Morgan). Luckily, the issue of where we would live was a no-brainer as we both felt that Mount Morgan was our only option as that was where our family and support systems were. We would go down to the cafeteria and browse the internet (using quite a few $2 coins in the process) and when we found something of interest, we would take Andrew down to have a look. We even made arrangements to view a house once we returned to Mount Morgan the following day. Time was of the essence and the type of property we were looking for weren't a dime a dozen!

Our Hell Week culminated in the family meeting we held

on our homecoming. We had made prior arrangements for all of our family to be at Andrew's parents so we could relay our story to everyone at once. To say that it was an emotional meeting is quite the understatement, but it was necessary. Andrew and I tried to convey our experience, but when it became too much, Rel finished communicating it for us. I so wanted to be strong that day. I wanted to be able to talk for myself, for us, and let people know that despite the diagnosis we were hopeful, thankful for their support and encouraged their enquiries. I wanted to let them know how we intended to go about things and that in spite of everything, we were doing okay, but I wasn't able to get it all out. Again, Rel's assistance was deeply appreciated and beneficial to everyone present as she was able to bring everyone up to speed and translate the medical side of things more effectively than I ever could.

Even though we were totally depleted following the epic family meeting, Andrew and I went and looked at a potential property. On seeing it and what it had to offer and considering the other properties available at the time, I was keen to sew things up straight away, without too much contemplation. Andrew wasn't quite as enthusiastic, but after debating the pros and cons, we made an offer on the property later in the day.

Change is Afoot

Sunday 24th of February

Returning home to Blackwater was like balancing on a double-edged sword. On the one hand, it was the greatest feeling to be home and surrounded by all things familiar, but on the other, it was bittersweet as we knew that our lives there and all that we had built, hoped, dreamed and planned was at an end. Whether we liked it or not, we had to leave the life we had made for ourselves in Blackwater and we were entering a new, unknown and uncharted future.

There was no escaping our new reality as we went to contract on the house we had inspected in Mount Morgan and made plans to have outstanding work completed at our place in Birt Street, have it subsequently appraised and put on the market as soon as practicable.

Things were moving at lightning speed, to the point where it was difficult to process everything. On top of Andrew's diagnosis and buying and selling houses, in the four days that we had at home, I had meetings with the kids' school advising that they would be leaving and I researched and enquired about alternative schooling options in Mount Morgan/Rockhampton. I resigned from my position at Tiny Tots Child Care Centre and Andrew and I attended meetings regarding his employment. I made appointments with solicitors, insurance companies, accountants, doctors, banks and financial advisors for when we returned to Rockhampton. Mindful of Andrew's condition, we completed what work we could on the house and made arrangements for remaining work to be finalised by others. We also received many phone calls and visitors as well as having the general tasks and duties associated with just being Mum and Dad.

I also started the laborious task of packing things up. Metaphorically, it was like I was packing up our old life and storing it in boxes with each item that was packed away. Our life was being reduced to a stack of boxes that were destined to be neglected and sit in a corner somewhere.

They say that it's not good practice to make significant life decisions or changes immediately after experiencing trauma as you would likely be prone to shock and your ability to make sound decisions could be compromised. Well, we pretty much obliterated the theory as we made enormous decisions within a very short timeframe following Andrew's diagnosis. With us though, it was more a case of having to than wanting to, as we didn't see that we really had a choice. Again, we didn't have the luxury of time.

Meeting with our friends and my work colleagues, who were also close friends, was onerous because not only did we have to relive our story over and over again, it was also the beginning of goodbye. Just as our lives were changed forever, so too were our relationships with others. Inevitably, the status quo within our relationships was upset, but for the majority this strengthened our ties and heralded much needed support.

With regard to our personal relationship, there seemed to be a gradual 'changing of the guard', in the sense that I began assuming more responsibility for things. Andrew had always been the 'doer' and the 'shaker', but because his condition didn't allow him to do what we both once took for granted, it was necessary for me to step up (although I don't pretend that I 'did' or 'shook' or handled a drill quite like he did). This was quite tough for both of us to assimilate because it was different to the way we had always done things. While our bond was fortified, our roles were blurring and neither of us liked it overly much. It upset Andrew to relinquish certain aspects of his role, but I think it hurt him even more that I was taking it on.

How easy it was for us to lie in our bed and pretend that the last few weeks hadn't happened. We played out this fantasy quite a bit, but the escapism didn't last long and coming out of it generated much discussion, of the sort that is not your usual breakfast fodder. One thing to come from these moments though was the revelation that our relationship could and would survive without all the fluff and glitter that we all seem to accumulate. It was all down to the ugly truths, but our commitment to one another was never in question. Despite everything, knowing that we were in it together, no matter what, was a good feeling to have.

Even though our time in Blackwater on this occasion was only short, it was very intense and physically and emotionally exhausting. Being away from our main support system (for the first time since Andrew's diagnosis), especially in relation to the medical aspect of it, was very frightening. Thankfully, aside from the constant presence of his symptoms to date and extreme tiredness, there were no major episodes whilst we were away.

The pace of things didn't slow down once we returned to the Mount. If anything, it increased because we had to attend all the appointments that we had set up while in Blackwater! We were quite practical about what things needed to be done and we tried to reduce the impact of doing such things by approaching them in a matter-of-fact manner. This didn't always work, but we tried. Andrew had always been very pragmatic about certain things and I had never been more thankful for this trait than now, especially in relation to work-related issues and insurances. He always thought ahead and when Hudson was born, he insisted on taking out separate insurances to those offered through his employment. He considered it a necessary evil and he liked to be prepared — for anything.

We only stayed at the Mount for a few days before going back to Blackwater. Prior to leaving, we attended a family barbeque at the Big Dam, celebrating Rel's daughter, Tay's birthday. While we enjoyed such gatherings, it was also difficult because the difference in Andrew's interactions and input into such affairs was all too obvious.

Over the coming weeks, we were back and forth between Blackwater and the Mount. During one trip to Blackwater, friends came around to visit us in the 'green beast', a Ford XY sedan. This used to be one of Andrew's projects, but they were well on the way to finishing what he had started. Despite not having driven for quite a while (he had made the decision to cease driving, which for Andrew was monumental, especially considering I was now in the driver's seat), Andrew took the 'green beast' for a cruise. He was absolutely knackered when they got back because there was no power steering and it took all his strength to keep it on the road, but he had an enormous grin on his face. Something I'd not seen for a long time.

Tuesday 4th of March

Some other friends made the trip from Yeppoon to take 'the ute' off our hands, another Ford XY. This was one of Andrew's pet projects and it had been on the burner for close to fifteen years! Given his love for the car, it was quite difficult for Andrew to give it up, but he was happy to know that it was going to someone that would appreciate it and do it justice, so to speak. When they were removing it, Andrew couldn't help but get amongst them, telling them where bits and pieces were and offering tit-bits of information about it. Although it was sad for him, it animated him and it was nice to see him with mates, joking around as though he didn't have a care in the world.

Quite a few of Andrew's mates took the time to visit, which he deeply appreciated. Like us, there was a general consensus of disbelief that the infallible "Panda" could be unwell, let alone have such a disease as Motor Neurone. In some ways, talking with others about what was going on and how we were dealing/coping with it was very confronting, but at the same time, it made us acknowledge and deal with what was happening.

While Andrew wasn't one to indulge, I arranged for him to have massages and Bowen Therapy during our stints in Blackwater. They offered him some relief, but left him very tired. He spent the majority of his time camped out in the lounge — thank goodness for Pay TV! — but he would always push himself to do things. When Sue and her husband, Wayne, came out to help with some work on the house, Andrew couldn't help but get involved. It was very frustrating for him to sit back and watch others do things and even though he would pay for it later, he pushed himself beyond his limits quite regularly. With regards to my packing up the house, Andrew would insist on helping and often became cross because he wasn't able to do as he wanted. To alleviate this, I tried to do most of the packing while he was otherwise occupied.

Thursday 20th of March

This was a pretty big day for us, for a few reasons. We'd made the trip in to the Mount the day before, but on that Thursday, we went to Rockhampton to drop off the contract for the sale of our home to our solicitor, meet with the Rockhampton Grammar School re Lainy attending next term (there was no place available for Hudson so he would have to attend the Mount Morgan school in the meantime) and we met with our bank. The most significant happening of the day though came around 10pm. I remember being a little fragile and sitting at the bar at the Nugget Hotel when Rel came out from the office and said that she'd found something that could be the answer to our prayers. After scouring the internet on and off since before Andrew's diagnosis, she kept coming across a doctor in India who specialised in embryonic stem cell treatment. On researching the matter further, information provided about the treatment seemed to be just what we were looking for.

For the first time in a long time, we were energised and very hopeful and after sharing the information with Andrew, he was the first in line to say 'why the hell not!' The following day, Good Friday, Rel emailed Doctor S. about Andrew and much to our surprise and relief, she answered later that same day. She requested as much information as we could provide and asked that we make a video of Andrew showing and explaining his symptoms. We did this immediately (by no means an easy feat) and after having the video converted and emailed, we eagerly awaited a response.

Saturday 22nd of March; my birthday

It was my birthday on Easter Saturday and while I'm always quite spoilt (because all birthdays are very special), I was even more indulged this year. I received gifts that I will treasure for my lifetime, from my *I love you always* t-shirt to my gold heart pendant with Andrew's and my initials on it. There were more than a few tears shed because for some reason, the significance of the day (for me) seemed to magnify what was happening one trillion-fold.

We spent the remainder of my birthday and Easter at Mum and Dad's partaking in all the hoopla associated with the bunny festivities. We made Easter baskets, bunny footprints and cotton ball trails and staged the traditional Easter egg hunts. Again, the emotional roller coaster was in full swing, because along with the joyfulness that such times of the year and get-togethers bring, they were interlaced with the ever-present oppression that seemed to shroud us.

Monday 24th of March

We returned home to Blackwater the same day that it was decided that Andrew would venture to India to undergo the embryonic stem cell treatment. Once more, we were thrown into chaos because never before had we travelled overseas and so had to initiate the process to procure the necessary documents and the like to enable such travel to occur (example: passport and visa). It was also established that Andrew couldn't make the trip alone and while I was desperate to go with him, I knew that this was too selfish of me because the kids would also need me, given that we would be moving and they would be changing schools and such. This was one of the many times I faced the dilemma of wanting to be in two places at once! While we all had the same sentiment, it was decided that Rel and Gav would be the two who would accompany Andrew.

Planning for their trip promptly began and given the time-frame we had set ourselves — two and a half weeks — things were frantic. Apart from having to wait for the necessary documentation and make relevant travel arrangements, we liaised very closely with Doctor S. in India regarding the treatment Andrew would be receiving and the logistics of his stay once the team arrived in India. She operated a Hospital as well as a Clinic, both located in New Delhi. Initially, it was planned that Andrew's treatment would be administered over a three-month period. While our decision for Andrew to undergo the treatment never wavered, the fact that he would be away from all of us, especially the kids, for such an extended period of time was of grave concern. We considered time to be precious, but we truly believed that Andrew's time with us could be extended, by his undergoing the treatment. Rel and Gav also had to arrange leave from their respective employment and make familial arrangements to accommodate their absence.

With all the frenetic madness going on, including packing, cleaning, planning and organising, we still tried to attend to the normal, everyday things, especially in relation to the kids. We went to parade, school disco's, had kids over to play, facilitated sleep overs, visited the park and went to barbeques, one of which was a going away gesture for us, which was touching, but quite sad as it highlighted our predicament. As far from normal as things were, we had to have a semblance of normality, for the kids' sake, if nothing else.

We had an enormous amount of help in the moving department. Friends offered to do all manner of things for us. Some brought a huge stack of moving boxes and one came with a truck load of wood shavings for the garden as they knew we were selling the place and wanted to help spruce it up. Others took ute and trailer loads and in some instances, truck loads, of gear for us. While we were going through the process of purchasing the place in Mount Morgan, we stored quite a lot of our stuff at Mum and Dad's in the interim. It was very convenient for us that Dad had such a big shed!

Sunday 30th of March

Andrew and I went to the Mount as we had business to attend to in Rockhampton the following day. The kids stayed with friends in Blackwater overnight, but we were home in time to pick them up from school Monday. Whilst in Rockhampton for our lightening quick visit, we called on Real Estates to put our other property in Glendale on the market; went to the solicitor to lodge Power of Attorney documents and finalise a settlement date for the property at Mount Morgan; completed and lodged school forms for Lainy and as Rel had booked the flights for India (departing 12th of April), we arranged travel insurance for Andrew (which was quite difficult given his health status) and picked up other travel paraphernalia so the task of 'packing' for India could begin.

Mum and Dad also came out to Blackwater on the Monday to

assist with our packing and everything else involved in moving. Additionally, they helped out with the kids, which freed us up to concentrate on other things that required our attention.

Whilst I wasn't to accompany Andrew to India, it was planned that I would join them in mid-May for a few weeks (and my sister Tan would travel with me). By this time, I was hoping that the kids would be somewhat settled in their new environments at home and school. Again, my desire to be with both Andrew and the children was relative and regardless of which way I went, there was guilt because I couldn't be everywhere at once, even though I knew it was irrational to think I could be! Wanting to be everything to everybody was very taxing and while you know it is impossible, it doesn't stop you from wanting it or feeling inadequate because you can't do it. The gaping hole of emptiness that was once my stomach churned constantly with guilt, inadequacy and fear and by no account is it a combination I would recommend.

Wednesday 2nd of April

Rel flew to Brisbane to personally lodge her, Gavin and Andrew's visa applications for India as she was advised that this would be the most efficient way and it would expedite the process. It was also the last day that Hudson, Lainy and Andrew spent in our house in Blackwater. We had a parade of visitors all day, wishing us well, saying goodbye and some were more than generous, leaving us with personal treasures to help our plight or just give us comfort. That night, I remember all of us lying in our bed and we were talking with the kids about moving and why it was necessary when Lainy asked 'when Daddy would get better?' Immediately, Andrew and I locked eyes and shared a pained moment as we tried to fight our own fears and emotions and find the words to explain that we didn't know if Daddy would get better. This is definitely one conversation I wish never to experience again.

Merle and Roy came out on Thursday to pick up Andrew and the kids (although they didn't escape the cleaning/packing frenzy as I put them to work!). After having ice-cream parties at school as a final farewell to their classmates and friends, the kids climbed into the car with their Dad and grandparents and said their last goodbye to the only home that they had ever known. Saying goodbye to them all was harder than I imagined, even though I knew I would be seeing them in a few days' time. It was enormously lonely being at home by myself, knowing that the place would never again know the presence of Andrew or the kids. I was bereft and even more saddened to know that Andrew wasn't doing too well either, emotionally or physically.

My last night at home was spent cleaning the kitchen, with the help of one or two bottles of red wine. It was quite surreal being in the empty house by myself and I remember seeing Andrew everywhere I looked. He was in the cupboards in the kitchen where he chose their colour; in the slump glass window that we put in place of the old front door; in the entryway where he had built in the veranda; in the patio that he had built just before Hudson was born; in the bathroom where he had installed the new vanity basin and even in the loo where he had picked out and installed the throne. Our house in Birt Street was very much a part of Andrew as he had quite literally put a lot of blood, sweat and swearing into it. It was very hard to say goodbye to our house for many reasons, but none more significant than it having been the only home that our children had ever known.

Saturday 5th of April

Moving day. It started early and while I expected the familial troop to arrive and assist with the move, many of Andrew's mates showed up to help out as well. As busy as I was and with all the chaos, I couldn't escape the fact that this was it and after giving the floors a final mop, I wasn't quite brave enough to take one last look around as I feared it would be my undoing. In closing the door that last time, I was doing more than saying goodbye to our home. I was officially closing the chapter on our old life — our happy, not-a-care-in-the-world, life. Again, as I drove out of Blackwater with our two dogs, Tank and Josie, and the car loaded up to capacity, I couldn't make myself look back in the rear-view mirror. I probably wouldn't have been able to see anything through my tears anyway.

I recall telling Andrew, following our move from Gum Street to Birt Street in Blackwater that I would never, ever be moving again. Thankfully, with all the assistance we received, the task was less painful than it could have been. I should also point out that I was very fortunate in the unpacking stakes as I didn't have to do any of it! There were an army of helpers on hand to do the dastardly deed for me and I didn't even mind that I knew where nothing was. I figured I would find whatever needed to be found when I needed it.

The next week was taken up with the business of settling in to the Mount, packing for India, receiving Andrew, Rel and Gav's travel visas and transferring the money for Andrew's treatment, sorting through housing issues, building a temporary enclosure for the dogs (thank you Uncle Tony; Rel's husband), getting things organised for the kids' schooling, rest, good quality family time and some much-needed retail therapy. Mum and Tan also gave me a heart-shaped pendant that had a picture of Andrew and I emblazed on it, with the kids on the other side. It remains close to my own heart always and is one of my most precious belongings.

Wednesday 9th of April

On the first night in our new home, Amanda (Moo, Fan's daughter and our resident photographer) came and took some family photos. Andrew was totally wiped out by the end of it (and he wasn't one to get photos done at the best of times) and I'm very sorry now because we never actually took individual photos of the kids with Andrew. While Moo suggested it, I said not to worry about it as Andrew was too tired. We should have taken the time because even though they are only photographs, a picture says a thousand words.

The day before Andrew left was hard to get through and we were all fragile. We had visits from close friends and that night we all congregated at Merle and Roy's for a send-off dinner. It was lovely to have everyone together, but again, it highlighted the importance (the desperation) and the hope that we all had pinned on them going to India and what it would mean for Andrew; for all of us.

India – Take One

Saturday 12th of April

I'm pretty sure I didn't sleep the night before they left. I just lay in bed touching and looking at Andrew beside me; thinking, hoping, wishing. He didn't get much sleep either as he was up before the alarm. As they were on the 6:30am flight, we had to leave the Mount at 4:30am. Even though it was ridiculously early, a few others came to the airport as well to see them off. I tried to be strong and not let Andrew know how hard it all was for me, but he knows me well and could read it in every line of my face. I guess we were trying to be strong for one another, but I'm not that good an actress.

The scene at the airport could have been out of a Mills & Boon novel; not that we were concerned by anyone else's thoughts or presence and we could only wish that what we were experiencing was a work of fiction. I wanted to be close to Andrew through every step and after checking in, we sat and waited until it was time. We said little, but communicated a lot. We never actually said good-bye, but I was able to tell him I loved him and to stay strong and positive. I wanted our last hug to go on and on because I couldn't bear to let him go and while Rel assured me they would look after him, letting him go was very, very, very hard.

Despite his own emotional anguish and the physical pain that he was in, Andrew forwent the allocated wheelchair and walked out to the plane and to our astonishment, climbed up the stairs. His determination was shining through and it was almost like he was sending us a message through his actions, letting us know that he was fighting. Seeing Andrew board the plane and watching it take off did nothing but intensify the vast emptiness in my chest and the ache in my heart. It was almost a physical pain. Knowing that I could only be with him in spirit was a harsh reality and even though I had no doubt that Rel and Gav would stay true to their promise, not being there to share everything with Andrew and support him myself was really tough.

After a very long day, Andrew called at around 10:30pm to let us know they had arrived in Hong Kong and again at 9:30am the next day to say they were in India (approximately twenty-five hours travel time, including the four-and-a-half hour time zone difference). A diary was started on the day they left to record the happenings and allow all of us left behind some insight into all that was going on. (While this was the diary's primary function, it also served as a tool of remembrance and allowed us to track Andrew's illness as we kept it going on their return.) Gav was the initial author and amongst all the detail, there was a large dose of humour. The diary entries certainly elaborated on the stories/occurrences we shared during our many phone calls and all excerpts from said diary will forthwith be depicted by italicized text.

Regarding our travel to India, the service provided by the airline, Cathay Pacific, was very accommodating and they provided for all of Andrew's needs. By all accounts, the Hong Kong airport was massive and we had to catch a train within the airport to get from the arrival to the departure gate. We were suitably impressed with a young female airline worker whom simultaneously pushed Andrew and another person (for what seemed like kilometres) in wheelchairs, leaving Narelle and I (Gav) eating dust. We concluded that she was on steroids or in training for the 2008 Olympics...or both! If Hong Kong was the 'Myers' of the airport world, Delhi Airport was definitely the 'Franklins'

— certainly No Frills here. In fact, words can probably not describe what we were all thinking/ feeling at the time, other than maybe — "What the F!K are we doing here!"*

We walked out of Customs to a sea of onlookers holding up signs for pick-ups and thankfully one was for us. We headed outside where we were groped and pleaded with by beggars wanting to carry our luggage, which we tried to ignore. We knew this would happen, but seeing is definitely believing. We were put in one car and our luggage in another, which made us a bit nervous. Nevertheless, we set off amongst the overpowering smog, the 'make the rules as you go' traffic, punctuated by beeping horns and incessant flicking of lights. We were glad to get to the clinic, which was quite nice, especially compared to what we had just driven through. Once settled, the guys slept for a few hours and later that morning, one of Doctor S.' colleagues came and conducted a very thorough physical examination of Andrew and obtained a history of his symptoms and their progression.

Monday 14th of April

It was all systems go as Andrew had his initial face-to-face meeting with Doctor S. She was extremely positive and radiated hope, all the while collating information relative to Andrew's case and focusing on the future. Andrew was started on medications to assist with his treatment and he had a physiotherapy assessment (as this would play a large role in his overall treatment plan). Doctor S.'s medical partner, Doctor A., met with Andrew later that afternoon and administered his first dose of stem cells intra-muscular (I.M.). As there was no adverse reaction, a program was to be formulated and the regime was to begin the following day.

Half a world away, things were also progressing at a rate of knots. The first day that Andrew received his full treatment of stem cells, was also the first day that Hudson attended Grade One at the Mount Morgan Central Primary School. Housing and legal issues were still being sorted, the last of the unpacking was being completed, permanent dog pens were being constructed (and none too soon as Tank was often getting out and wandering to the neighbours!), I was battling Telstra with regard to internet coverage and Lainy was getting ready for her first day of Prep at the Rockhampton Grammar School.

We talked nearly every day on the phone and sent text messages, exchanging information and filling each other in on what was happening. Even though Andrew was thousands of miles away and had more than enough to occupy his mind, he wanted to know the ins and outs of everything that was happening at home. Sometimes though, Andrew would be too tired to talk or he would only be able to do so for a very short time so Rel and/ or Gav would let us know what was going on. When Hudson was named Student of the Week, Andrew sent a congratulatory video message, which the kids loved and we received a few photos of Andrew.

In addition to the stem cell treatment (which Andrew was receiving I.M., intra-venous (I.V.) and via infusion, Andrew was having daily physio, participating in yoga when he was up to it and due to his oxygen saturation levels, had to concentrate on his breathing exercises, all of which he found exhausting. During one physio session, Andrew reported witnessing a miracle. We met a quadriplegic who had been on a respirator for fourteen years after breaking his neck during a footy match from a spear tackle — fourteen years to the day! We all witnessed him breathing by himself for the first time without a respirator. Doctor S. said it was the world-first case of this happening. Pretty exciting stuff! We were meeting people every day with similar stories. Even though it was a hard slog and each person at the Clinic had their own tale, Andrew (and the others) drew strength from such stories or 'miracles' as they fuelled feelings of hope.

A few days before Gav was due to leave India, the inevitable happened — Delhi Belly. Surprisingly, Andrew wasn't too badly affected, but Rel and especially Gav were suffering. The diary entries for this period were light on, but the story of Gav literally diving from the bathroom to the bed and not knowing how you could be that sick without dying always brings a smile (and when Gav gives an animated recount; giggles).

Sunday 20th of April

Gav left India and later said it was very hard to leave Rel and Andrew behind knowing what he was leaving them to. With Rel taking over diary duty, she noted on Monday that she received a text from Gav. *Made it to Brisbane airport okay, thank god. When I left him at Delhi Airport (where the sign says International Standard Airport — what a joke!) I was made leave him at the entrance by guards with guns (scary). That was an awful feeling, not knowing if he got onto plane or not, thank Christ he's home.*

Once Gav was gone, it was only Andrew and Rel and while they had each other, they were so far away from the rest of us. The distance didn't seem quite as far when there were three of them. Apart from everything else that she was doing, Rel was on a mission to find Andrew some real food as nearly everything on the menu was curried — even the vegetables and the rice! With the assistance of some of the Clinic staff and an upstanding tut-tut (scooter taxi) driver, Rel sourced some steak and prawns, which they enjoyed immensely. She even purchased cooking utensils and was playing master chef until her little outfit was shut down due to 'safety' reasons. This probably wasn't a bad thing after her 'chicken man' experience! On her travels, Rel found a shop selling fresh chicken — literally. Following her order, a live chicken was picked out, killed, plucked and it was almost too much when the man put the chicken on the cutting board and he himself joined it! He had a knife in each hand and each foot and he proceeded to cut up the chicken. Rel surpassed mortification and was unable to accept the chicken offered, even though the man had gone to all that trouble — her tut-tut driver ate well that night!

Concerned with Andrew's restlessness, difficulty sleeping, lack of food intake and general well-being, Rel spoke with Doctor S. and requested that stem cell dosages be increased so as the treatment time-frame could be reduced, thus allowing them to return home sooner. It was further established that Andrew wasn't tolerating the environment (especially the smog and food) and while there wasn't anything that could be done regarding the former, Andrew's diet was changed so as to not include any curry or spices and he was also receiving regular I.V. fluids to ward off dehydration and supplement his diet. Doctor S. considered Rel's arguments and Andrew's dosage was subsequently increased so he was receiving four times the dosage per day. It was also decided that Andrew be prescribed a mild sedative to help him sleep.

Rel attended a Clinic meeting along with the other residents, carers and the doctors. It was unfortunate that Andrew couldn't attend (as he was too unwell) as everybody shared their stories, which were a great inspiration. Doctor S. also explained how the stem cells are grown and collected. From conception, the embryo cell takes fifteen days to become a foetuscell. She collected the cells before the fifteen days so the cells have no D.N.A. or memory and they grow and divide. She explains that it's like being pregnant for nine months then the cells have to reach milestones. As such, recipients are not allowed to do anything that a pregnant woman can't.

Friday 25th of April

While Hudson and Noah marched in the local ANZAC Parade, Andrew started a new, world first, protocol. *It was planned that for the next ten days, Andrew would receive a certain (enormous) dosage of cells per day — more than any individual has ever had at one time. We can book our flights out for May 5th. Gav and Linda onto it. Well, he has had stem cells in every orifice; mouth, lungs, muscles and veins...Not only is he having I.V. and I.M. cells, he had them on his tongue and nebulised into his lungs. Wow, what a body filled with babies we're going to have to nourish.*

Tan's and my jaunt overseas was not to be as Andrew and Rel were now expected back prior to our departure date. There was no disappointment regarding this though as I'd much rather have Andrew home. To change their flights was another matter entirely as it couldn't be done at our end. Thus, Rel had to venture out and find the airline office in Delhi, placing her trust (and extra rupees!) with a stranger. The ordeal took a number of hours due to the location of the office and both Andrew and Rel were extremely anxious. Essentially, both of them were alone in a foreign country and the prospect was alarming, to say the least.

Saturday 26th of April

Given Andrew's health status, Doctor A. asked Rel if she should take him home. She advised that flights had been booked for the following Sunday, but they would leave earlier if necessary. *Andrew really wants to hang in and have his cells. Can't blame him so would I. It's a bit tough but we'll be okay...Not a good night. Andrew can't breathe real well. Shallow when sleeping therefore wakes himself up when deep breathes. Quite distressed during the night. Rang Gav. We're going home. Need to sort out his breathing then look at coming back. Flights arranged. Will leave early in morning, Jet Airways.*

The one constant thing in our lives is change! Didn't sleep a wink, too scared that alarm won't go off...Hard trip to Singapore. Andrew very unwell. Jet Airways moved us up to first class. Andrew had oxygen and was great. Singapore to Brisbane not good. Full plane. Finally made it to Brisbane 6:50am and guess who was picked to open bag for Border Security? Yep, me!

While it's not obvious from her diary entry, Andrew and Rel's trip home was worse than horrendous. Andrew was quite literally incapable of doing anything, given his tiredness, lethargy and inability to breathe and he was totally reliant on Rel for everything. The strength of them both is astounding and the fact that they both made it home came down to their shared determination and unwillingness to give up.

Home Again

Tuesday 29th of April

Gav and I caught the red-eye to Brisbane and planned to meet Andrew and Rel at the International Airport, but just before the train from the Domestic Airport to the International was due to leave, Andrew rang and said they were already at the Domestic. As wonderful as it was to finally see them and have them back, both Andrew and Rel were beyond exhausted as neither had slept for days. We could practically see the relief on their faces that they had made it this far, but we had another stint to go and while it was only an hour flight to Rockhampton, it seemed to take forever. Andrew's breathing was of grave concern as he was using his ancillary muscles to breathe — each breath was a huge effort for him and took considerable energy. I sat next to Andrew on the flight to Rocky and even though he was desperate for sleep, he would only close his eyes for a few seconds before waking up because he would stop breathing. It was freaking me out, so I couldn't even imagine what it was like for him, or for Rel who was a witness to it for so long and powerless to do anything about it.

We took Andrew straight to the hospital on our return to the Mount, where he received oxygen and fluids. Given his condition, it was decided that he would remain in hospital, not that I think he would have cared where he stayed as he was so tired. The kids (and everyone else) were overjoyed and very content now that Andrew was home and they had seen and talked to him. Gav stayed the night with Andrew and reported that he had some good stretches of sleep and I'm becoming more convinced that

Rel is part machine as she didn't leave the hospital until late, ensuring that Andrew was settled before she would go.

Wednesday 30th of April

Andrew felt a little better the following day, although he was still very tired and sapped of all energy. He alternated between the oxygen mask and nasal prongs (that also provided oxygen) and whenever he went without the oxygen, he felt short of breath. Rel contacted Andrew's Neurologist and he in turn made contact with a Respiratory Specialist at the Prince Charles Hospital and the decision was made that Andrew go to Brisbane that day. Arrangements were made for Andrew to travel via Aerial Ambulance due to his health status as it was obvious that he wouldn't be able to go commercially in his current state. I flew out of Thangool (just outside of Biloela and the flight was delayed!) and Rel and Al were to follow the next day.

On arriving in Brisbane, I went to the motel and then onto the hospital and as I was waiting for Andrew to arrive, I realised that my anxiety levels had not decreased at all in having Andrew home. If anything, they were rocketing. It was very frightening and confronting sitting in the hospital waiting room and that's what I did — waited, waited, waited, until Andrew arrived around 1am. He hadn't enjoyed that flight one little bit as he had to be restrained on the trolley. Given his inability to breathe and the fear of choking (as he was lying down), not being able to move was nearly unbearable for him. A sentiment that Andrew shared with Rel and Gav, prior to his leaving Rockhampton in the plane. One could imagine their anguish at having to let him travel alone.

Even though it was early hours of the morning when Andrew arrived and was admitted to the hospital, there was no rest as he was visited by numerous doctors and subjected to various tests (such as blood gases — blood samples taken from an artery to test the level of oxygen in one's blood). We dubbed one of the doctors 'The Jabber' as he had quite a few tries to extract the blood, but failed. Thankfully, the next doctor was more successful. The results of these tests were very concerning and warranted a visit from one of the Respiratory Specialists in the very early hours of the morning.

The Specialist advised that the blood gas results were alarming as normal CO_2 levels should be between forty to forty-five and Andrew's level was around sixty (and another Respiratory Specialist later pointed out that such levels were indicative of Andrew being in second degree respiratory failure). The Specialist asked a barrage of questions and further alluded to our 'future plans' and basically encouraged us to get our things together and 'have the chat'. Not being prepared for such a consultation, its impact was substantial. Already being afraid out of my wits, our talk with the Specialist nearly put me (and Andrew) over the edge. We did talk after he left, but it was more to comfort one another than anything else.

The Specialist returned a short while later with a BiPAP (Bi-Level Positive Airway Pressure) machine and after explaining how it worked as a form of non-invasive ventilation (with preset levels of inhalation (IPAP) and exhalation (EPAP) pressure levels relative to the patients' needs, it provides positive pressure when breathing in and lowers the air pressure when breathing out), he fit Andrew with a face mask, fiddled with the levels and following this, Andrew was able to breathe. By the time Rel and Al arrived at 8am the next morning, Andrew had seen four doctors, had numerous blood tests and observations and he had been using the BiPAP for about an hour.

Initially, Andrew was fighting the machine, but once he became used to the mask (which covered his nose and mouth), he relaxed and let the machine do its job — Andrew was able to sleep for the first time in days. Given his poor condition, Andrew was assigned a nurse, one-on-one. He was constantly monitored.

Once Andrew was settled, Rel stayed on and Al and I went back to the unit to rest. During our absence, the doctors visited again and information was shared regarding Andrew's stem cell treatment and his current condition. According to Andrew, the doctors were all 'doom and gloom' and he said, "they had me one foot in the pine box...gone in six months." Following the discussion with the doctors, Rel had her own discussion with them outside and new understandings were reached and Andrew's requirements regarding the cells were heeded.

After a period of time on the BiPAP machine and some much-needed sleep, further blood gases were conducted and results showed that Andrew's CO_2 levels had reduced considerably. The doctors appeared to be amazed by Andrew's response to the machine and indicated that they had not seen anyone recover like he had. They conceded that a large part of Andrew's condition was due to exhaustion.

Friday 2nd of May

While Lainy participated in rehearsals for the signing choir, Andrew's Neurologist and the MND Nurse visited us at the hospital. During their visit, we discussed the viability of Andrew having a Percutaneous Endoscopic Gastronomy (P.E.G.; feeding tube) inserted to assist with his nutritional intake (as it was clear that he was not sustaining on his current diet alone. The process of eating was absolutely exhausting for Andrew and as a result, he wasn't eating a lot. Thus, his body wasn't getting enough fuel to counter the excessive energy that was being expended through such basic functions as breathing and eating — things we all take for granted and don't give a second thought). As the procedure would likely be necessary in the future, we weighed up our options, given that further risks would arise (re anaesthetic and such) as Andrew's respiratory system became less effective. Despite the risks involved, Andrew didn't really hesitate in giving his consent for the procedure to be performed and arrangements were made for it to occur as soon as possible.

Andrew was visited by the Resident Speech Pathologist and the Physiotherapist. The latter did stretching exercises and took Andrew for a walk down the corridor. They later returned with a wheelie walker and recommended that Andrew start going for little walks starting tomorrow to try and build himself back up and increase his mobility and strength after having spent four weeks in bed.

There was no denying that Andrew's health had improved since being admitted to the hospital and he indicated that he was feeling tired, not exhausted, which for us, was a huge distinction. However, he felt that being on the BiPAP was making him short of breath and we deduced that it was because when he was using the machine, he was receiving adequate breaths/intake and when he came off it, he wasn't receiving as much. It was going to take time for his body to readjust to a) having sufficient oxygen and gas exchange while on the machine and b) coming off the machine. Further breathing tests were also conducted and it was noted that there were significant differences from when Andrew did the same tests in February. There was also no denying the reduced function of his diaphragm muscle.

Andrew had quite a few visitors throughout the day and Rel had to return home, but planned to return when Andrew was due to have the P.E.G. procedure. Both Al and I decided to stay with Andrew at the hospital and while some of us didn't have too much trouble sleeping (it was established that I don't do night-shift very well at all!) Andrew was quite restless, but doctors wouldn't authorise a sleeping tablet for him due to his compromised breathing.

On Saturday, Andrew was feeling pretty shattered, but he had periods where he felt quite okay. During one of these periods, we did Andrew's physio and he showed us what type of exercises he was doing in India. He was tired out by the physical exertion and we decided to forgo the wheelie walk as he didn't want to overdo things. Al and I stayed at the hospital again and the chairs we converted to beds were surprisingly comfortable.

Sunday 4th of May

Even though he didn't really want too, Andrew made himself go for a wheelie walk through the ward. He found it much easier to breathe when he was walking and pushing down on the walker's handles and he took off like a rocket! The exercise really tired him out and he did little for the remainder of the day. His spirits were brightened though as he had some visitors.

There seemed to be a pattern emerging with regard to Andrew's sleeping habits as he would go on the machine two or three times during the night and would have his best sleep in the early hours of the morning. He tired around 9am and would go back on the machine for one or two hours of rest/sleep. One of the Respiratory Specialists came in and talked with us about the BiPAP machine. It wasn't a very joyful or uplifting discussion, but they apparently have to give the spiel to all those who utilise the machine. He basically advised that it was not suitable as a long-term option.

Even though things were quite dire, Andrew didn't lose his sense of humour and he thought it hilarious when I freaked out because I thought he was choking on one of his tablets. His giggles were forgotten later in the day though when the boy who cried wolf really did choke, twice! We had another visit from Andrew's Neurologist and we went for another wheelie walk, but Andrew wasn't keen to go downstairs and venture outside.

As the P.E.G. procedure was scheduled for Tuesday, Rel and Sue came down the afternoon before. Staff from the Sleep Lab also came on Monday to try Andrew with various face masks and he went into the Lab to spend the night so he could be monitored. Rel stayed with him.

Tuesday 6th of May

Things started off well as Andrew had slept from 11pm to 5am — the longest sleep he's had in weeks, possibly months. To prepare for the procedure, Andrew had to have a special shower and to my delight, a shave as the masks seal better when he's clean-shaven. Andrew wasn't overly thrilled by his theatre garb, but I thought the hat and purple gown were very fetching.

True to form, the procedure was delayed and Andrew didn't go down until close to midday. We had to attend the endoscopy section of the hospital and to get there, we had to traverse the 'tunnel' or the bowels of Prince Charles. It was quite surreal going from the ward to what felt like the underground. On leaving the tunnel, we had to go from one building to another and in the process, we passed through sunlight. It was the first time Andrew had been out in the sun in a long time. Rel and I had to stay in the waiting room and it was almost like deja vu as Andrew was once again going somewhere that I couldn't go with him.

After a very long and anxious wait, Andrew returned from theatre and we learnt that the procedure could not be performed due to the location of Andrew's stomach (it was too high due to the weakened muscles and diaphragm). We were all gutted, but none more so than Andrew. The Respiratory Specialists visited and we contacted Andrew's Neurologist and discussed our options. It was proposed that Andrew have a nasal-gastric tube inserted, monitor to see whether it's viable with the mask, return home for four weeks so he can recover and recuperate, then return to have the P.E.G. procedure conducted radio-graphically at the Royal Brisbane. While not overly keen on trying the nasal-gastric tube, Andrew consented to the plan.

Once the plan was finalised, we set about organising BiPAP machines for when we went home (we decided we would need two machines, using one as a backup). Rel and Al returned home that night and Fan and Stacey (her eldest daughter) visited. Apart from their visit, it was a pretty crappy day!

Andrew had the biggest sleep so far on the machine — from 10:30pm to 7:30 am Wednesday, 7th of May. Despite this, he didn't feel overly refreshed. To further mar his day, nurses came to put in the nasal-gastric tube. Things didn't go well and in the end, Sue ended up putting it in herself. Andrew absolutely detested it and his gag reflex was working overtime. He was prescribed Maxilon to relieve the gagging and he didn't even flinch at the needle. Once the tube was inserted, Andrew needed to have an x-ray to determine whether it was positioned correctly, which it was. The matter of removing the wire from the tube was complex and in the end, Sue rang Rel and she basically relayed information as to how it needed to be done. The nurses were under pressure to perform and to their relief (and Andrew's), it finally came out. Andrew persevered for about three hours, but couldn't tolerate the tube any longer so he had Sue pull it out. He said that out of everything he had experienced thus far, the tube would have been the worst.

To counter some of the trauma of the day, Andrew had quite a few visitors and while my aunts, Tricia and Fran, were there, Sue and I went back to the unit for showers. On returning to the hospital, staff provided Andrew's prescription for the BiPAP machine and I went off to pick up the second machine from their depot (the hospital were lending us one in the interim). Much to my chagrin, the taxi driver advised me that I must have a 'difficult life', which I took to mean I must have looked pretty damn awful. On top of this revelation, the company didn't have the proper machine, but I took it anyway! During my absence, Andrew had visits from the Social Worker, Physiotherapist and the Dietician who recommended that he up his intake to 4200 calories a day. Fan and Stacey also visited and spoilt us with Sue's favourite — divine white chocolate-coated doughnuts.

Thursday 8th of May

Andrew had a sleep in on Thursday morning, but on waking, he still felt tired. Despite this, he was as excited as the rest of us because we were going home. Prior to this, we decided to purchase our own BiPAP machine as it seemed to be a lot less hassle than renting and it would give us peace of mind. Following yesterday's debacle of ordering one machine and getting another, we figured it was worth the $100 cab ride to collect the new machine ourselves and it was worth it to know that we were getting what we ordered. The hospital was providing us with a second machine (our back up) and while we had the outdated machine that we picked up yesterday, we decided to take it home with us as well as we didn't have time to return it. We would send it back once we were home.

Andrew wasn't overly hungry, but he had some lunch and not too long after we started our journey home. He had no energy whatsoever so we wheelchaired him to the taxi and once we arrived at the airport, QANTAS provided us with great service. Once through security and in the waiting lounge, Andrew went on the 'Turbo Charger' (BiPAP) for about half an hour to recoup from the trip from the hospital and to get ready for the flight. The plane trip to Rockhampton wasn't too bad, but Andrew found it harder to breathe due to the higher altitude.

Rel picked us up from the airport and took us home. Once we

were home, it was quite emotional because a) we were relieved to be home and b) we were happy to be home and having the family welcome we did meant a lot. It was also great to see the kids and just be together again.

Understandably, Andrew was pretty shagged from the days' events so we tried to make him as comfortable as we could in our bed. It wasn't ideal, but we were hoping it would be a satisfactory interim measure as we had ordered a 'you beaut' Enterprise 8000 bed (which Andrew had had in hospital) and it was due to be delivered on Monday or Tuesday. The bed had been a godsend whilst Andrew was in hospital as it allowed you to move the back or leg sections any which way and it was easier to find a comfortable position. While the beds were only on trial at the hospital, we knew we had to get one for Andrew at home. His comfort level was our only consideration.

During our absence, Merle and Roy purchased an electric lounge chair for Andrew (one that lays totally back or stands up, assisting one out of the chair). We were also loaned a wheelie walker and various bathroom chairs.

While Andrew and I were very happy to be home, the kids were especially happy to have our little family reunited.

Andrew's appetite seemingly increased with our return home, which we were all happy about, but we were mindful of the types of food he had. His diet consisted mainly of soups, vitamised drinks and high calorie juice poppers as they required less energy for him to ingest and they decreased the risk of his choking. We whipped up a mean milkshake (protein enriched and extra ice-cream), but Andrew soon became tired of them. This didn't stop us from trying to make him have them though. All in all, Andrew had quite a good weekend, despite the ever-present tiredness and lack of energy.

Monday 12th of May

This was a big day for Andrew in terms of visitors. In addition to the usual, a friend and fellow Lodge Executive made the trip in from Blackwater and some other relatives also visited. While Andrew seemed to enjoy such visits, I fear they were difficult for him in the sense that it was hard for him to allow others in to see how things had changed; how he had changed. Most persons who wanted to visit would contact first and the decision to see them was always left up to Andrew. We used to talk about this quite a bit and I recall saying that this was our life now and this was who we are and if people weren't comfortable with that, for whatever reason, that was their issue.

As the 'Enterprise 8000' (the super bed) was due to be delivered the following day, Monday night was the last night we had in our bed. It was going to be good-bye king and hello king-single, for both of us. Thinking back now, it was literally the last night that we slept beside one another in the same bed — such precious memories.

To our amusement, 'Startrack Express' delivered the 'Enterprise 8000' and we weren't even Star Trek fans! It was all systems go as we had to disassemble our bed and remove it before the other could be brought in — through the window! It was quite a feat as it was enormously heavy, so we were thankful that we had a few extra hands to help us out. We had the bed on the back of Roy's tilly and he backed up to the house and we put it in through the window as it was too big to manoeuvre through the hallway and door (this became an issue later on as we realised there was no accessible doorway to get Andrew and the bed out of the bedroom, should we need to in an emergency. We contemplated various contingency plans from the ridiculous: pulling him out on blankets, to the extreme: remodelling the room and putting in a bigger doorway).

Once Andrew's bed was in, we put in my Gran's old bed (Skinny Winnie's single) so the rest of us would have somewhere to sleep. During its time in our room, Gran's bed gave quite a few injuries thanks to the sharp edges of the end bedposts. It left few unscathed and we soon covered the offending posts to minimise damage to ourselves. While I wasn't fussed on Gran's bed (in comparison to my own, much bigger bed), Andrew was very happy to have his special bed and at last he was comfortable! He was able to move the bed himself via the head panels and we could move it from the main panels located at the middle of the bed. The kids thought the bed was great, but it wasn't without fault as not all of the panels worked! Surprise. Surprise.

Wednesday 14th of May

This was the day Tan and I were due to leave for India, but she left for home instead as she'd been visiting for a few days. The M.N.D. Nurse also made contact to see how Andrew was travelling and to discuss the possibility of his joining the M.N.D. Register. She forwarded information regarding the Register for Andrew to have a look at.

Thursday saw Lainy catch the afternoon school bus from The Rockhampton Grammar for the first time. It was quite anxiety-provoking, but her older cousins, Tay and Georja caught it at the next stop and shared the adventure. Andrew being Andrew, he was always thinking of the future and planning so we started the paperwork for his various Total and Permanent Disability (T.P.D.) insurances and contacted his employer and various doctors' relative to the claims. We also had contact from the Prince Charles Hospital, as the Respiratory Specialists wanted to follow up with Andrew when he returns to the Royal Brisbane for the second attempt at the P.E.G. procedure.

Sue stayed over and slept in with Andrew on Thursday night.

As someone stayed in with Andrew each night (for company or just to be on hand if he needed anything or the machines played up) we often had others stay over. During the initial stages, I usually stayed in with him and the others would come and give me a break, but as time went on and Andrew's needs increased, the nurses of the family (and sometimes Fan, my fellow assistant-in-nursing-in-training) took over the majority of the nightshift or we shared. Sometimes there would be three of us, plus Andrew. It was like one big slumber party and it wasn't unusual for one of us to sleep in the walk-in-wardrobe!

We were also in the habit of doing Andrew's physio on a daily basis, usually late in the afternoon/night. We followed on from exercises that he had been given by the physio in Brisbane and India and we made up a few of our own! We would have liked Andrew to see a physio more regularly, but it wasn't feasible as he wasn't really able to travel and few would make the trip to Mount Morgan for sessions. The next best thing — us, and we became pretty good at it. We would concentrate mainly on his feet, ankles, legs, shoulders, arms and hands and a full session would last anywhere from half an hour to an hour, depending on how he was feeling and what he could tolerate.

Over the next few days, we booked for Andrew to return to the Royal Brisbane on the 3rd of June, he received numerous visitors and Gav hurt his back and spent quite a bit of time at home convalescing with Andrew. We also made attempts to weigh Andrew as it was obvious that he had lost an enormous amount of weight. Prior to his illness, he was around 110-115kgs and while it wasn't a truly accurate reading, we surmised he was now around 90kgs. Such a dramatic loss over a short space of time highlighted the importance of Andrew having the second P.E.G. procedure (and it being a success) to ensure that he was receiving adequate nutrition. In addition to this, it was imperative for the cells survival.

Given Andrew's waning condition, we felt that it would be much better for him to receive any further treatment at home (in Australia) as opposed to his travelling overseas again. In an effort to make this happen, the Therapeutic Goods Association (T.G.A.) was contacted and after talking to several persons regarding Andrew's circumstances, paperwork was forwarded for us to complete. It appeared that nobody really knew the process as a request to import embryonic stem cells had never been made previously. Pioneering again!

Further to his condition, it was necessary for someone to be with Andrew at all times. Thus, when Lainy had her eisteddfod performance and both she and Hudson had their respective sports days, others had to cover my absences. So not only were we reliant on our family for their support at night (in terms of sleeping over), in getting the kids to and from school, doing general everyday tasks like grocery shopping or picking up the mail, they helped out whenever I had other commitments. I considered myself very lucky in the sense that I was able to go out if I needed to. Andrew didn't have that luxury.

Wednesday 21st of May

This was not a particularly good day for Andrew as he wasn't travelling very well, physically or emotionally. Despite visits from a few good mates, his demeanour didn't change and it was further exacerbated by his not being able to get comfortable or fit his mask properly. He quite literally said that he'd had enough and for the first time, was openly angry and animated. It was a hard day for all of us, because we all wanted to comfort Andrew and make things okay, but none of us could. Watching his anger, pain and inner struggle was heart-wrenching, especially because we too felt helpless.

The gloom didn't lift overnight, but was further fuelled by

Andrew's having to shower (which was extremely taxing) and his nearly choking, which also drained him physically as well as being absolutely terrifying, for all of us. Whilst recovering, we did receive some happy family news — Jamie and Jodie (Rel's son and daughter-in-law) were going to have a baby. Andrew and Jamie shared a very close bond and on finding out, Andrew was joyous (but I also feel he was anguished because his future was so uncertain and eight to nine months was a very long way away). I guess we'll never know whether his few tears were due to the former or the latter.

We received information and paperwork regarding the M.N.D. Register and Andrew's T.P.D.'s, so this occupied our time for a period while we filled out the various forms. We also followed up with the Prince Charles Hospital re Andrew's booking for the Royal Brisbane. Jamie had also been organising for us to have a shed constructed and they poured the slab on Friday. We thought it a great excuse to get Andrew outside for a little while and even though I made stacks of immovable black marks on the walls with the wheelchair on the way out, it was worth it to see Andrew outside, talking to the guys and having input into what was going on.

As we had feared, the skin on Andrew's nose broke from the constant friction and pressure from the mask. It's just what we didn't want, but given the amount of time he wore the mask, it seemed inevitable. As it was necessary for him to continue wearing the mask, we devised many methods of covering the broken skin and trying to alleviate his discomfort and we used a trial and error process to see which was the more effective option.

Saturday 24th of May

The kids and I were banished from home as 'The Unit' had a sleepover at our place. We left home just after lunch and spent the afternoon with Gav's wife, Thorlene and her crew and we had our own little sleepover at their place. 'The Unit' came prepared; bringing enough food and goodies for ten sleepovers, but the primary motive of their gathering was to spend some quality time together. It was also tentatively planned that they discuss certain matters with Andrew regarding 'worse-case scenario', but this didn't eventuate as Andrew was too unwell and not in the right frame of mind. They did manage to get him outside and even though he wasn't feeling the best, he enjoyed their congregation and company immensely.

As it was Roy's birthday the following day, everyone came to our place for breakfast and most came back for dinner as well. Andrew was exhausted from yesterday's events and his glum mood continued, although it seemed to pick up during visits from friends throughout the day. Regarding this however, he was very good at masking his true feelings when he wanted to and it wouldn't have surprised me if he purposely 'put on a happy face' for their benefit.

With the dawning of a new day, Andrew's mood also seemed brighter. He was more interactive and quite jovial at times and his being happier impacted positively on all of us. Irrespective of this, his food consumption continued to be of great concern as his tiredness was further limiting his intake and he was getting very tired of the shakes! A scheduled visit by the Dietician didn't occur as she was under the impression that Andrew already had the P.E.G. in. A phone consult ensued and by all accounts, there was little else we were able to do, although she did suggest he have a few more shakes!

Andrew made the comment that his limbs felt weaker and he was becoming unsteady on his feet. While we encouraged (or his take on it: nagged) him to go out to his chair in the lounge, Andrew was spending more and more time in the bedroom as he was more comfortable in the bed and he didn't have to be as mobile. As good as he was at manoeuvring the wheelie walker, it was becoming more difficult for him to walk.

Tuesday 27th of May; Gav's birthday

It was Gav's birthday and our house was full again as everyone came out for a celebratory afternoon tea. Andrew often said that he much preferred the house full of people to the quiet and it seemed to reflect in his character as he was having a relatively good day, was more positive and was even making jokes. The fact that we had a big flat screen TV wall-mounted in the bedroom likely had something to do with his good mood as well! We also tried to make Andrew's bed more comfortable by putting a doona under the sheet and he received a massage in an attempt to alleviate some of the soreness in his back.

Tuesday was also special because the application for the importation of the stem cells was completed and only required the local doctors' signature before being sent off and there was a story on the local news station about the fellow in India who breathed without his respirator and his embryonic stem cell treatment for a spinal injury. Some of the footage that was shown in the story was taped while Andrew was in the same hospital room in India. We were all quite excited about the story due to the exposure it was providing and this story was followed up the next day with the story of another person with a spinal injury undergoing the treatment. Again, Andrew had also met this person whilst in India.

When Andrew woke up on Wednesday, he said he felt the best he had for a long time. It was great to hear him being so positive, but the mood of the morning soon changed as Andrew fell on the way out of the bedroom. His foot caught on the carpet and his left leg/knee didn't lock in and he fell down. It was an effort, but we pulled him back up and into a chair and while he was unhurt from the fall, apart from some carpet burn, the incident absolutely exhausted him and it was necessary for him to go onto the machine to recuperate.

The application for the stem cells to be imported into Australia was sent off and people from the T.G.A. contacted the Mount Morgan Hospital later that afternoon and made arrangements to have a phone conference the following day to discuss the application.

As Lainy was catching the bus home from school on Thursday, the fate of our application was decided. Approval to import the cells into the country was denied due to the "moral and ethical" debate surrounding embryonic stem cells. Our disappointment at the outcome was extreme and despite valiant argument by Rel and Andrew's Doctor, the T.G.A. didn't waver from their decision. Given that the cells couldn't come to us in Australia, we now had to consider Andrew making another trip to India. Not an easy decision and one that wasn't made overnight.

In addition to the application being refused, our power went out for nearly three hours. This caused concern given our dependence on power for such things as Andrew's bed, chair and the breathing machines and while we survived without incident on this occasion, the importance of having power available to us was highlighted. Dad went home and returned with a generator — better to be safe than sorry. Needless to say, I had a training session on generators. We also had a few visitors and as Andrew was quite stiff and sore in the back and shoulders, he had some massages to relieve the kinks.

Friday 30th of May

After Andrew's morning routine, his face and neck were covered with red blotches. It was caused from the CO_2 build up, but after a short period on the machine it righted itself and he felt okay. Andrew was in a positive mood and was quite the jokester throughout the day. It was great to see him happy, although it was counteracted by the fact that his legs were shakier and he was finding it harder to breathe when standing up and it was increasingly difficult for him to find a comfortable position in bed that allowed him to just lay there without his mask on. All of these things were of enormous concern to us, but he valiantly carried on and entertained guests to boot! One of his visitors brought him a Brucey's pizza (best bite in Blackwater), but his other gift of a St George hat that had been signed by some of the guys Andrew worked with was the real treat. He loved it.

It was a time for visitors as Andrew received a few more in the ensuing days. One of which was a close colleague and he presented Andrew with a Commemorative Saint George watch from his specific crew. It was quite an emotional moment. We were also humbled by the receipt of a donation from the Blackwater Rodeo Committee, which was totally unexpected and the gift of a willow tree Angel — the Angel of Hope, from one of Andrew's aunts and uncles. Whether they were worth a lot or a little, to us it didn't matter; they were priceless as it showed that we were not alone.

Tank (our male pug) even tried to get in on the action, coming in and climbing up onto Andrew's chair. He just went crazy! He jumped all over Andrew and at one point had his butt against Andrew's cheek, which Andrew thought was hilarious. Andrew must have mellowed, because he thought the red marks, welts and putting up with the doggy smell were worth it for the pleasure he obviously got out of it.

Given that we were going to Brisbane on Tuesday, Andrew had a late shower on Monday, before he went to bed. It proved to be a bad idea as he was so tired. We had difficulty in getting him up and out of the shower and trying to manoeuvre him around the shower screen was not at all easy. It wasn't a comfortable night; not for any of us as we didn't really know what to expect from tomorrow.

Always Waiting

Tuesday 3rd of June

Lainy went off to school as normal, but Hudson was quite upset when we left for the airport early on Tuesday morning. While the travel itself was extremely taxing on Andrew, the ongoing movements from car to wheelchair to plane and so forth were exhausting in themselves. This, coupled with the fact that we were delayed by fog was a recipe for disaster. By the time we arrived in Brisbane and presented to the hospital, Andrew was totally spent. It didn't help matters that the nursing staff had no knowledge of our arrival and we had to meander through the admission process. One familiarity though, we were given the same room on Ward 7B North as we had on our last visit. Given that this was the 'room' where we received Andrew's diagnosis, I'm sure we were all hoping that the ambience and outcome would be a little more cheerful and positive this time around.

We were advised that the dictating factor in Andrew's undergoing the procedure (to have the PEG inserted) was whether there was a High Dependency Unit (H.D.U.)/Intensive Care Unit (I.C.U.) bed available. True to form, there was nothing free on the day of our arrival, so we would have to WAIT! Not something that we do well, although Andrew was absolutely ravaged by the days' events and was very weak and in need of rest — as were the rest of us.

While Andrew had an okay night, the appearance of one of the Doctors the following morning advising that the procedure being conducted was dependent on the availability of an I.C.U.

bed, did not bode well. Again, we were waiting and while he could ill afford it, Andrew was nil by mouth, just in case the procedure were to eventuate. Whilst waiting, we had a visit from various Doctors and the Palliative Care Team. While we are sure they are lovely people in their own right, we didn't take kindly to the connotation of their visit and this extended further to the doctor that arrived to advise the procedure wouldn't be going ahead today. We were told that it would be happening first thing the following morning and we were provided with the 'shower pack' so we could have Andrew up and ready, first thing in the morning. Meanwhile, he was still 'nil by mouth' and very weak, considering he'd not had any substantial intake for a number of days. At one point, Andrew was given a small dose of morphine to see whether it alleviated his breathing difficulty, but it didn't seem to have any noticeable effect. It was debated whether it would be beneficial for him to have a slow release dose after the procedure.

We were at the hospital very early on Thursday morning to help Andrew shower with the special pack and get ready for the procedure. To make things a little easier for him, we experimented by having the machine in the bathroom with us so he could continue to use it during the process. It seemed to have the desired effect as Andrew coped well, although it was a little tricky trying not to get it wet.

After his shower, we waited and waited and waited and waited. Finally, the Specialist came in, but it was to advise that the H.D.U. continued to be full and wouldn't allow for Andrew's accommodation. Thus, the procedure would not go ahead today. Saying that we were upset and cranky is an understatement! We shared our displeasure as Andrew had essentially been waiting for three days, during which time he had been nil by mouth! How much longer would we need to wait? How much longer could Andrew wait?

While we were waiting, I made arrangements to fly home the

following morning. As much as I wanted to stay with Andrew, tomorrow was Lainy's fifth birthday. Torn again — having to choose one or the other. As much as I wanted to stay with Andrew, we felt that one of us needed to be with Lainy on her special day. I didn't have any qualms that he wouldn't have the best support crew in my absence and this was my saving grace on many occasions and made my decision to return home a little easier to bear.

As we continued the waiting game, Sue arrived and some ladies from admissions came to finish up some paperwork. Unbeknown to us, one of the ladies' names was 'Jan' and whilst they were in the room, Gav vented and during his tirade he came out with, "Not happy, Jan!" We didn't realise this until after the ladies had left and we all had a good giggle about it. That poor woman, goodness knows what she thought!

We again brought it to the staff's attention that Andrew hadn't had anything for three to four days due to the procedure being delayed and his being nil by mouth. They made arrangements for the I.V. team to come and give him some fluids, but before they arrived, Andrew was taken down for the procedure. Finally! It was around 3:40pm.

We didn't wait well. Gav and I continued our 'eat off' and we went to the H.D.U. waiting room... to wait. Andrew's Neurologist visited and we thanked him for being our advocate. We also had visits from my aunts' and one of our nieces. The anxiety in the waiting room was intense and while we all tried to stay positive, it was sometimes too big a task. It was a very scary time. At one point, we talked about the cruelty of M.N.D. and how it was inherently on-going (especially for Andrew) because of the deterioration of the body, but continual soundness of the mind. We also talked about how difficult it was to be an observer and watching what the disease was doing to Andrew and being powerless to do anything to stop it. The tragedy of people dying unexpectedly (such as car accident victims) was also discussed and to my horror, in some respects, I thought it would be easier because at least there would be no long-term suffering, at least not for those who die.

Andrew was brought to H.D.U. around 5:30pm and the procedure was successful. We were so relieved. Understandably, he was extremely sore and very tired, but as always, with the little strength that he had left, he was assuring us that he was okay. He was hooked up to an array of monitors and there were wires attached to him all over the place, but to me, he'd never looked better! I stayed with Andrew until Gav came to do the 'night shift'. The staff in the H.D.U. were great. They allowed us to care for Andrew and only intervened when necessary.

As funny as it sounds, being in the H.D.U. with Andrew and being surrounded by the trauma of the place, we shared some very special moments. Just being together, holding hands, looking at one another — some very special moments.

Friday 6th of June; Lainy's birthday

It was very hard to leave for home the following morning considering Andrew was still in H.D.U., but I couldn't not be with Lainy on her birthday. Sue kept us up to speed on Andrew's condition, letting us know that he wasn't transferred back to the ward until late in the afternoon and he was feeling very sore, very tired and very weak. Andrew stayed on the machine all day and they began feeding him through the P.E.G. While he wasn't well enough to travel, he was ultra-keen to get home.

Saturday was a big day on many fronts. Andrew came home in the morning and by all accounts, it was a shocking trip. According to Andrew, it was nearly worse than coming home from India! To make matters worse, the car adapter we had for Andrew's machine blew a fuse so he wasn't able to use it on the trip to the

Mount. As a result, the car ride home was very, very fast. I was in such a state, I didn't even realise I didn't have my seat belt on until after we got home!

While happy to be home, Andrew was very weak and dehydrated. He also stayed on the machine all day as his tummy hurt when he was off it due to the effort it took him to breathe.

Jamie and co. started putting the shed up and there was a "Panda Golf Day Fundraiser" held in Blackwater, which had been organised by some of Andrew's mates. Humbling. Dad ventured out to Blackwater with Hudson and Lainy and attended on our behalf. The community response to the fundraiser was unbelievable and we were totally blown away by everyone's support.

While Sue stayed with us on Saturday night, Rel and Gav came out Sunday morning to help get Andrew up and do his routine. Our plan was that one of them was to be present all the time and at least one of them would come out in the morning and night for his routine.

Andrew had a bad night, suffering from wind and the mask was annoying him. We got him comfortable in his chair in the lounge and as he was so dehydrated, he ended up having two and a half bags of fluid! We had the drip attached to a coat hanger and set up on a picture hook! I imagine it looked a sight. Andrew stayed on the machine for most of the day and at one point he had a small dose of morphine. Luckily it was only small, because he had an allergic reaction!

The kids were ecstatic to see Andrew when they got home from Blackwater and the feeling was mutual. They didn't seem to be concerned at all about Andrew's PEG and after some initial curiosity, they accepted it for what it was.

Given that it was becoming increasingly difficult to manoeuvre Andrew in the bathroom, we decided to remove the glass shower frame and replace it with a curtain. Wayne (Sue's husband) started the process by taking out the glass and Jock (Fan's husband) was called on to make some aluminium ramps for easier access with the shower chair. We're fortunate to have such handy men around.

Monday 9th of June

Today wasn't a good day. While Andrew appeared to be getting stronger, his P.E.G. was infected and required antibiotics and he was on the machine nearly all the time as the effort of breathing without it was painful and the pulling of muscles irritated the P.E.G. site. He was simply tired of everything. He had had enough! It was very disheartening to see him so negative and it was hard to respond to.

Andrew was having feeds every hour and he had another bag of fluids, although his lack of output was concerning. He had blood tests to check his kidney and liver function and thankfully, the results were okay.

Given everything that was going on, Sue made the decision to stay with us for two to three weeks.

During Andrew's morning routine on Tuesday he had a shower. He did really well considering he did it without the machine and having a mobile shower chair and no glass hampering our movements made it a lot easier.

They had a piece in The Blackwater Herald (the local newspaper) about the Golf Day held at the weekend and it was accompanied by a story about Andrew. Wow. It was odd reading about ourselves in that context and a little disconcerting knowing that everyone else was reading it too. Not that we'd ever hidden what was happening, but seeing it in print was quite confronting.

Throughout the course of the day, Andrew was a little emotional at times, although he seemed more positive than the day before. During one of these moments, we cocooned ourselves in the bedroom and took some time out.

Apart from it being Jamie's birthday and Queensland winning the first State of Origin, Wednesday wasn't that fabulous. Hudson was unwell and home from school and Andrew had had a really bad night.

Andrew couldn't settle or get comfortable and didn't get a lot of sleep as he felt the machine was lagging and his mask was becoming claustrophobic. We contacted the Doctors at Prince Charles Hospital about the machine and they indicated that a blood gas test needed to be done to establish levels and see whether the machine settings needed adjustment. The Director of Nursing (D.O.N.) came out to our place and did the test and the levels were quite good. We considered the possibly of anxiety being a factor in Andrew's breathing difficulty. Despite the perceived lag, Andrew remained on the machine for most of the day as he felt he couldn't get a proper breath without it.

Andrew didn't feel too bad on Thursday morning and he went off the machine for his morning routine. He's become physically stronger and is able to move more without assistance, although he still had trouble lifting his arms.

We completed some paperwork regarding Andrew's T.P.D.'s and I purchased the BiPAP machine and some accessories. We also had contact from Lainy's school to say that Hudson would be able to attend there next year, which we were very happy to hear. Josie (our female pug) was also creating a concern and needed to be taken to the vet. In amongst all of this, we had some quiet time. It was nice, just being us and we savoured the time, but we both thought it was also nice to have the house full of people.

What Now?

Friday 13th of June

We certainly weren't disappointed as the day and date lived up to its reputation. During Andrew's morning routine, he had acute abdominal pain on the right side and it got progressively worse until he was vomiting from the pain. When the pain didn't subside, the doctor came out to see him and Rel contacted the Neurologist. After discussions, a urine test was conducted and confirmed that Andrew had renal colic — kidney stones! Needless to say, we were stunned. In hindsight though, given his stay in hospital last week and his lack on hydration for an extended period, we shouldn't have been surprised by the outcome.

Andrew had copious amounts of Pethidine and some other medications to keep him as pain free as possible, but nothing took all of the pain away. An unexpected benefit of the Pethidine was Andrew being off the machine for most of the morning. He found it easier to breathe on his own and only had to use the machine as all of the medications he had were making him very drowsy. Andrew passed some 'calculi' late afternoon and once this occurred, the pain receded.

Despite the traumatic events of the day, Andrew didn't have too bad a night. However, at 5am the following morning, Andrew experienced similar pain on the left side! Surely it couldn't be? Yes. Yes, it was. Were we surprised? No.

Pain relief started early and while he'd had a huge amount the day before, it was nothing compared to what he was given today! Despite this, Andrew continued to experience some pain and it was an extremely long day. He was feeling very washed out and tired and the latter was the only reason he felt he needed the machine. For the most part, Andrew went all day without the machine. An unexpected correlation arose between the administration of Pethidine and Andrew's ability to breathe on his own.

Neither Andrew nor Sue had a restful night, but it didn't appear to have an adverse effect on his morning routine as he went through it without the machine. It included a shower and a shave and I'm thinking that maybe the pain medications decreased his anxiety of my having a razor at his throat!

The pain continued until late afternoon and only eased when Andrew passed some 'calculi'. Following this though, he showed signs of having the beginnings of a urinary tract infection, but the girls were on to it straight away! Despite not having had much food wise in the past few days, Andrew had feeds as normal today as well as drinking more water and having one and a half bags of fluid. He was totally bushed at bedtime, but he had enough left for a few giggles. Something so small, but meaning so much.

Andrew had a very restless and unsettled night. Despite trying lots of different things, he didn't really get comfortable until the very early morning and as a result, he had a sleep in. Once he was awake, the feeding assault began. Throughout the day, he had the most intake thus far, as well as having some lunch orally and two bags of I.V. fluid.

Given the events of the past couple of days, Andrew continued to be sore and have pain around the kidney area. Regarding this, he persevered with minimal pain relief as he didn't want 'hard' drugs today. He was also very tired and had no energy. He felt he had 'nothing' in his legs, arms and shoulders and the mask was proving to be problematic as well. His feet also remained swollen so we had to elevate them. During our physio session, we found a new shoulder stretch that seemed to work and brought Andrew some relief.

Tuesday 17th of June

We decided to try different drugs at different times to maximise their effect on such things as Andrew's sleep and alleviating his respiratory drive. He did try to go without the mask for a little while, but he really needed to work hard to breathe and it was too exhausting for him.

Around lunchtime, Andrew ventured out to the lounge. Over time, our bedroom seemed to be becoming somewhat of a sanctuary for him and he was coming out less and less. Given that this was where he was most comfortable it wasn't really surprising, but any outside sojourn was met with positivity and encouragement, as we didn't want him to be isolated from the goings on outside his little haven.

Andrew was back having regular feeds, but tests showed there was still blood in his urine, so he had a couple of bags of fluid to flush it out. Thankfully, the level decreased indicating that it was remnant from the trauma of the renal colic, not indicative of another episode. Sue did Andrew's physio while he was in his chair as he was so tired and didn't feel up to the works. I also contacted the Prince Charles Hospital to enquire about batteries for the BiPAP machines.

We had a few visitors and some friends called to see how Andrew was going. We also received a parcel from Resmed containing the converter to allow us to use the BiPAP in the car and we assembled a 'thank you' basket full of chocolates for the staff at the Biloela Hospital for all their assistance. Josie was also taken to the vet and needed surgery to have teeth removed!

Wednesday saw Andrew up and out of bed fairly early. All was not good, however, as the blood levels in his urine had increased overnight. Rel contacted a leading urologist and we were advised not to panic.

Some of Andrew's mates visited, which he seemed to enjoy. One advised that he and a few others were arranging a football match between B.M.A. and Curragh (mines at Blackwater) as a fundraiser for us. Wow. He told Andrew to think up a name for his team (B.M.A.) and some ideas for a jersey design. His wife also surprised me with a spa package from 'the girls', which was unexpected, but received with great appreciation. In some areas of our lives, we are truly lucky — good friends are precious.

Sue and I attempted to lure Andrew outside, but he wasn't keen and the weather wasn't co-operating, as it was pretty miserable. Dad brought up an electric wheelchair that a guy was generously loaning to us. We had a hard time keeping the kids out of it.

Thursday wasn't a particularly spectacular day. Josie ended up having seven teeth out and Hudson lost his glasses. It wasn't all bad though, as one of our friends visited and we watched a DVD of the Golf Day they held in Blackwater. We had quite a few laughs, but it was also very emotional and we shed a few tears. Again, having good friends and seeing that people genuinely care is humbling and overwhelming.

We're not sure exactly how it happened, but on Friday, Andrew strained a sheath muscle in his back and was in immense pain. He tried to move as little as possible and required regular pain relief throughout the day. It was also Lainy's last day of term and she became sick and had to leave early. Not the best way to start holidays.

Apart from Andrew's back pain (which was easing), the weekend was challenge-free as there were no new developments. We had some friends visit and I was able to take the kids to the movies.

Andrew continued to be on the machine most of the time, which wasn't ideal, but nonetheless necessary. While he had to be off it at times during his morning routine, the process seemed to be becoming increasingly exhausting and we noted that once finished, he had a red rash that sometimes reached as far down as his navel. It was likely a build-up of CO_2, but it receded relatively quickly once Andrew was back on the machine.

Monday 23rd of June

Today proved to be a very difficult and emotionally exhausting day, for all of us. Rel received a call from the Palliative Care Team in Brisbane and they wanted to know whether we had had 'the chat' with Andrew. Did we know what he wanted or where he was at exactly or were we transferring our desires/wants/needs onto his? I had been running errands and Gav caught up with me at the grocery shop, saying there had been a call and we needed to talk about some things. I felt instantly sick, but wasn't really sure what it was all about until we got to Gav's and Rel told us of the content of the call with Palliative Care. The sick feeling didn't go away.

We thought we knew what Andrew wanted, but the call made it necessary for us to literally 'have the chat'. I wanted to talk with Andrew initially, even though I knew it was a conversation that I didn't want to have and I didn't have the faintest idea of how to have it. As always, Andrew knew something was up with me as soon as I got home. I sat down beside him and we talked. We cried. We talked. We cried. I told him we all loved him and would do everything and anything for him; even if that meant letting him go, if that's what he wanted. Andrew said he was tired of the struggle, but he was not ready to give up yet.

The relief of hearing him say that was unimaginable. His courage would never fail to astound me.

Rel, Gav and Sue came out and we were all very emotional given the subject of discussion. It was tissues all around, but we established that Andrew wanted to continue the fight and we made plans accordingly; together, but with Andrew in control, as it has always been, but we had refined the process. Andrew knew we were there and would continue to be there no matter what and it was with this confidence that he made the decision to return to India for follow up stem cell treatment. He said he was going to try it all and give it everything he had because he wasn't ready to give up. In making this decision, he was literally putting his life in our hands. He trusted us.

While I hope never to experience one of these days ever again, the outcome was positive in the sense that we all seemed to have new energy and we knew the direction we were heading in was the right one for us. A word of advice though, I would encourage anyone with a partner to have 'the chat' or something similar regarding an individual's needs and wants, should it ever get to that point, before one of you is at that point. I understand it's difficult to know what one would be feeling at that time, but if there have been discussions previously, surely the process would be a little easier? Just a thought.

Not surprisingly, Andrew didn't have too good a night. He woke early, had some pain medication and slept quite well after. On waking again, he endured the ordeal of shower and shave before going out to his chair in the lounge.

The house was quite full throughout the day with everyone visiting and it was nice to be surrounded by everyone. Especially after the day we'd had yesterday. I made contact with Ergon Energy and arranged for us to be flagged as a priority, given our reliance on power for the BiPAP. Even though we had the generator as a back-up, it was better to be over-prepared than under-prepared. I also contacted Telstra and requested they prioritise our phone line.

Hudson melted my heart today as he asked me if wishing stars were real. He said if they were and he wished on a star, he'd wish that Daddy would get better. He also drew a picture of himself with Andrew and a sky full of stars. I told him that would be my wish too.

Wednesday passed without any new developments. I contacted the Prince Charles Hospital regarding batteries for the BiPAP and was advised that Resmed (maker of the machine) was bringing one out in the very near future. Resmed was contacted the following day and I ordered three units — one for each machine and a spare.

It was hard to believe that three weeks had gone already, but Sue left on Thursday (26th of June) to return to her own life and family, in the physical sense anyway. We are so lucky to have such selfless relatives! Before she left, she helped us to shave Andrew's hair. It had been annoying him as it was pulling with the straps of his mask so he decided it had to go. It was the first thing his mum noticed when she came out.

Andrew was feeling quite strong today and we could feel the difference when moving him about because he was helping out a lot more. We also changed the dressing on Andrew's nose. It was very angry and red, but the skin wasn't broken.

Planning for India has commenced! The trip over there this time will be monumentally different to last time given Andrew's increased level of need. As a result, we needed to be ultra-organised and have all scenarios covered to make sure we were as prepared as we could be. Everything needed to be planned meticulously to reduce the risk to Andrew.

Now that Sue had gone home, Gav and Al joined Rel in the 'sleep over' roster and Fan stayed every now and then as well. Sue said she'd be up as often as possible.

Friday 27th of June

Andrew remained in bed all day as he had severe muscular pain in his back. He had massages and pain medication to ease his discomfort, but he was not comfortable. We had a few visitors during the morning and in the afternoon, I escaped and went to Rockhampton to run some errands and take Hudson to get new glasses. As bizarre as it sounds, we think a bird took his last ones — strange, but true and a lesson as to why you don't take them off outside and leave them on the septic tank!

Andrew didn't have a good night, as his back was still very sore, requiring pain medication. He was also experiencing 'bathroom blues' which was adding to his discomfort. Exhausted from his lack of sleep and his morning routine, Andrew wasn't fussed on going out to the lounge, but once he was in his chair he was able to get comfortable. We had a few visitors during the day and Rel spoke with the Doctor, making arrangements for him to visit Andrew at home on Wednesday afternoons. Sue also came back today and stayed in with Andrew.

The dreaded shower and shave happened again on Sunday and as usual, Andrew was shagged afterwards. We had contact from some guys we went to school with which was nice and some of my relatives arrived for a visit. To our delight, Andrew had some soup orally at lunch as well as his usual feeds via the P.E.G. On moving Andrew back to bed, we put him in on the opposite side to see if it made any difference, but it didn't. His back pain was still present and he felt his muscles were tight, especially his calves.

Monday 30th of June; Merle's birthday

Today started off as usual with Andrew's routine, but things soon became chaotic as he started choking on phlegm. Al was at work and on receiving the call she flew to our place with a sucker from the hospital. It was a scary experience for all of us, but none more so than Andrew. To reduce the risk of the same thing happening again, we put Andrew on bisolven twice daily.

The battery packs arrived at Resmed and arrangements were made for them to be couriered to us as soon as possible.

While Sue had to return to Biloela, everyone came to our place for tea for Merle's birthday. It was good to have us all together and once everyone left, we had a laugh at Tan's expense. She went down the driveway to close the gate and was met by two beady eyes in the darkness. A big dog was just outside the fence and scared the daylights out of her!

Phlegm continued to create issues for Andrew during Tuesday morning's routine. Given his weakened muscles, it was very difficult for him to get rid of it by himself. One positive though, the bathroom blues he'd been experiencing over the last few days were relieved and he was much more comfortable.

The site around Andrew's P.E.G. was very sore and in a surprise attack, Rel got to it with an alcho-wipe! Andrew said a little more than 'ouch', but it cleaned it up and had the desired effect. To date, the P.E.G. food Andrew's been having is banana flavoured and he was happy to find out he now had a choice of orange as well. Sadly though, the orange was not at all appetizing, so banana it was!

The kids were in the middle of their holidays and while we'd not been anywhere, they seemed to be enjoying their time at home. They'd do their own thing, come in and out and help with this and that. Sometimes they wanted to help do Andrew's physio, give him a foot rub, help with his P.E.G. feeds or just sit with him on the bed or lounge and watch TV.

On Wednesday, we were advised that one of Andrew's T.P.D. claims was going to be honoured and given our circumstances, it would be paid now as opposed to later. This was good news. The battery packs for the BiPAP machines also arrived and running true to form, we found there to be no connections. Such connections had to be purchased separately. We likened it to buying a car and finding it to have no wheels. You can't use one without the other so we ordered the connections.

We had a few phone calls during the course of the day from friends wanting to catch up and the doctor made his first house call. Mum, Dad and my aunt went home, but everyone else came out in the evening for the second State of Origin and Queensland won — yay! Andrew stayed up and watched the entire game, but he was super tired by the time it was over.

Given the trouble that Andrew had been having with phlegm, we included using the sucker as a part of his morning routine. This proved to minimise the risk of choking and required much less effort on Andrew's behalf. This morning's routine included a shower and shave and most was done with the mask on. Gav and I were getting very clever and my skills with a razor were improving, much to Andrew's relief.

Mum and Dad were due to come back up today, but as my aunt wasn't feeling well with some type of flu, they thought it better to stay away. Merle also had a call from one of Andrew's mates that we'd not heard from for many, many years. He had only just heard about what was happening and wanted to see how Andrew was. Tay, Georja and Bryce (Sue's youngest) also came out and we set up a salon in the bathroom and dyed their hair. At one point or another, our place on Keimar Road seems to have had it all!

The Dietician made a home visit and was quite pleased with how Andrew was going. Medication wise, Andrew was also put on a higher dosage Fentanyl patch. The patch was designed to provide ongoing medication over the course of a few days.

While Andrew had spent the majority of the day in his chair, he went to bed early as water was spilled on him and his chair. The incident was quite comical, but Andrew didn't see the humour until much later after the fact.

Friday 4th of July

Luckily for us, it was without fireworks and unexpected happenings. We had a few visitors and a call from one of the Respiratory Specialists with concerns re the battery packs. Regarding this, as the connections had arrived and we'd conducted our own tests, we advised that they seemed to be working well. We also changed Andrew's PEG end after the last feed of the day and due to phlegm issues, he had three lots of bisolven. The kids and I stayed in with Andrew and they thought it was great having a sleep over in the wardrobe!

Andrew had visitors over the weekend and Sue and I went on the internet, doing some research on India in preparation for our trip. Rel, Gav, Sue and I were all going with Andrew. On Sunday, the kids and I had a day out, going to the beach and out for dinner. It was good to get away and spend some quality time with the kids, but the whole time I was away, I found myself wondering what was happening at home.

Not sure how it happened, but on Monday, Hudson broke his glasses. There was also a story about Andrew in The Morning Bulletin (the Rockhampton paper) regarding the Golf Day held in Blackwater. On the home front, though, Andrew was doing it a little rough. His nose was exceptionally sore due to the pressure wound and the constant re-adjusting of the mask was irritating and not helping matters at all. We had also acquired a lift (via the Biloela Hospital) and utilised it for the first time getting Andrew out of his chair. While it was good for him to have a stretch, the lift seemed to put a lot of pressure on Andrew's chest and it was very uncomfortable for him. Andrew much preferred Gav!

Andrew had a little lie-in on Tuesday. Lucky. It was a tough day for him. His nose continued to cause pain. He required significant pain relief to settle it, especially after we went at him with an alcho-wipe! Need to be cruel to be kind? Leaving everyone to it,

Sue and I went to Rockhampton for the express purpose of going to Flight Centre to arrange tentative bookings to India. Tentative being the operative word as we realised that there would likely be many changes before anything came to fruition. We also indulged in a touch of retail therapy — never let an opportunity pass — and we also sorted out some new glasses for Hudson.

Wednesday 9th of July

Today was a very busy day. We had discussions with personnel from the Sleep Centre (Prince Charles Hospital) re options regarding masks and it was recommended we try another type — the Liberty mask. Al picked one up for us in Rocky and when Andrew tried it out — BLISS. Worked like a dream and provided instant relief as it only covered the mouth (as it had nasal prongs). Why didn't we know of its existence before? A mystery! I also made contact with Ergon Energy re Priority Assistance, Andrew's Doctor made a house call, we discussed medical forms necessary for international travel, some close friends visited and Noah (Gav's boy) came for a play date. We also exposed Andrew to the sun; albeit through the blinds in the bedroom, but we took what we could get!

Things are never simple. Thursday saw us sending further information to our local doctor regarding information and forms required for our travel to India — and there were plenty (airline medic form; access form; BiPAP form). We also needed to fill out further forms to acquire Priority Assistance from the electricity company and we had issues with the company who we sent one of the breathing machines back to. Was there no end? Apparently not, as Andrew was generally unwell and only had two feeds all day. He was vomiting and I was in desperate need of Codral Cold Tablets as I felt something sinister coming on and could not afford to share! In amongst all this, we ordered a sucker machine, as it was obvious that one was necessary for our daily routine. We also had visits from some close friends who thankfully, took it all in their stride. Given the events of the day, we didn't do Andrew's physio and Sue and I both stayed in with him through the night.

Friday was another significant day amongst many others. Andrew had a relatively good night, but by 5:30am, he was vomiting and we didn't know why, how or what! At some ridiculously early hour in the morning, Sue and I were changing Andrew's masks and as I took one tube out and was plugging it into another machine — the machine stopped. Just like our hearts! SYSTEM FAILURE — RING SERVICE. We somehow got the other machine operational, settled Andrew and then plugged in the other hospital machine again and it worked. We wasted no time in contacting the Sleep Centre and after much in-house discussion, we decided that having an extra machine would be most beneficial. While Andrew wasn't sure, I figured it would be better to have it and never need it, than to need it and not have it! We discussed our concerns with the Palliative Care Team and also made contact with Andrew's Doctor for his input. Not surprisingly, Andrew spent the day in bed. He had company though, as Hudson and Merle watched footy with him and Lainy shared her news of losing her first tooth!

Surprisingly, Andrew allowed the kids to take a picture of them together -one that will forever be a treasure. It was also a big day, in terms of the doctor having filled out the necessary medical forms for air travel, the letter written re Andrew needing BiPAP, Telstra Home Priority Assistance being approved and for Rel and Sue to have access to Andrew during our plane flight/ trip to India. While all this was going on, Andrew was having staggered feeds — 100ml at a time, which seemed to work well. Furthermore, one of Andrew's Lodge Executive mates made contact and told us that everyone in Blackwater was sending their goodwill and wishes our way. What a boost! He also said he and the rest of the Executive were planning to visit in the not too distant future. This buoyed Andrew's spirits, but it was also tinged with sadness.

What a weekend! I was under the weather and kept a very low profile, staying away from Andrew. The times I couldn't, I was garbed up to the max with a scarf wrapped around my mouth and nose — luckily the fashion police were nowhere around! To further ensure I kept my germs to myself, I was encased in a haze of Glen 20! Lucky Sue and Rel were on deck. Enough of me, Andrew had a relatively good weekend, although he stayed in bed. We kept him well hydrated (via bags of fluid), he was having normal feeds and his nose was on the mend, thanks to the relief provided by the new mask.

Andrew ventured out to the lounge on Monday even though he was extremely comfortable in the bedroom. We did some stretches while he was in his chair (and more later, once he returned to his bed) and he ate some stew without any dramas.

Tuesday 15th of July

Hudson returned to school and Lainy lost her second tooth! We received the second machine from the Prince Charles Hospital and although it didn't have a humidifier, we were happy it had arrived. Andrew had been using the Liberty mask, but it was hurting his lips so we swapped it for the Quattro, but it was hurting his nose — he just couldn't win! We filled out the medical form for Singapore Airlines ready for Rel to take to Flight Centre tomorrow — our trip was that much closer. Andrew's Power of Attorney had been registered, enabling Rel and I to legally sign on his behalf. Legalities regarding the kids were also finalised for when both Andrew and I were out of the country. We also brought a laptop in a bid to relieve some of Andrew's boredom — he surfed the net, played cards and chess and we joined Facebook.

Lainy and Hudson were both back at school on Wednesday and I had a parent/ teacher interview with Hudson's teacher in the afternoon, around the same time the Doctor made his house call. Gav wasn't around so Kenny helped us with getting Andrew up and down. He was very sore in the shoulders, was vomiting and after his morning routine, Andrew decided to stay in bed instead of going out to his chair. We did extensive stretches (especially with his arms), although Andrew continued to feel stiff and sore. As there were to be possible power outages throughout the day, we hooked up the batteries to Andrew's machine just in case.

One of the doctors from Prince Charles called regarding concerns with utilising the BiPAP on our trip to India. Apparently, there was no information pertaining to performance of the machines during flight. Thus, travelling with the BiPAP via plane was unprecedented and as a result, the hospital would not recommend or endorse the use of the BiPAP in this manner. We counter advised that we had acquired batteries for the machines and had been using them without incident.

Rel handed in the medical forms to Flight Centre and was advised that we would find out about flights to Brisbane by Friday. We also had the computer delivered, set it up and Andrew played a little chess and some cards, although using the touch pad was somewhat of a challenge — just one more to add to the list.

Flight Centre called on Thursday with the news that Singapore Airlines declined our travel as Andrew would need to be off the machine during take-off and landing. We provided further information regarding the machines, they were going to forward this information and try alternative airlines. In addition to this bad news, doctors from Brisbane called with concerns regarding Andrew's medication and how/amounts/when it was being administered. Well! I was glad to be out and unavailable when they called — Sue and I were in Rockhampton — so Rel and Gav spoke to them. Really, it's not like we were doing and giving him whatever we wanted, when we wanted!

Andrew didn't have a particularly good day either. He had a really sore throat (mainly due to using the sucker), the Liberty mask was hurting his nose, he was nauseous and he didn't venture out of the bedroom. Al and Fan stayed for the day and had a sleep over.

Friday was an enormous day for Andrew. We had quite a few visitors — some close friends, the Union Executive and two Palliative Care Nurses made their first visit. Re the latter, they indicated that Andrew should go to Rockhampton to be assessed as we were technically through the Brisbane Palliative Care, but this would unlikely occur until after our return from India.

The sucker we had on order had not arrived and was not even in the country so we were scouring the internet for a replacement. Not much success considering it was late on a Friday afternoon! Rel talked with Andrew's Neurologist and we also had contact from Flight Centre re they were sending forms for Cathay Pacific for the doctor to fill out.

Saturday 19th of July

During Andrew's morning routine, we had lots of drama. His machine turned off a couple of times because the battery connection was not secured properly! Needless to say, it was a stressful time for all of us. Andrew also had a shower, which added to his discomfort and not surprisingly, he remained in bed for the day. Due to the soreness of his nose, we were also alternating masks quite regularly.

Tan and the kids came to visit, Moo came up and brought some pictures of our family on canvas (which were gorgeous) and I took the necessary travel forms for Cathay Pacific to the doctor for him to fill out.

Our place was like a carousel with people coming and going.

On Sunday, Tan and the kids and Sue went home while Mum and Dad and Gav and Noah came to stay. We also had some friends visit for a few hours.

Following Andrew's morning routine, it was obvious that two or more people were required, as you needed extra pairs of hands. However, regardless of how many people were involved, the routine itself was very taxing for Andrew and he required time afterwards to recuperate.

On a more positive note, Andrew and Hudson decided on a jersey design for the upcoming football match. Hudson has been so excited to help Andrew choose the outfit (mainly red and white, with a 'V' as a nod to Saint George and flames) and Andrew had been happy for Hudson to have the majority of input. A real bonding experience for them — truly cherishable memories.

We had a very early start to the next week as Andrew had phlegm issues and subsequent vomiting at some ungodly hour on Monday morning. Later in the day, we were very happy to hear that Lainy was the 'Star of the Week', so that put a smile on our faces for a while. Andrew's didn't last long though because after some gentle (or not so much!) persuasion on my part, Andrew went out to the lounge for the afternoon. It was great to see him out of the bedroom, but I don't think he was convinced that it was a good move.

We ordered another sucker, which, of course, was much more expensive than the first, but we figured, why the hell not. We needed one and why not get the best? Dad dropped off the Cathay Pacific forms to Flight Centre and we emailed them information regarding the sucker (as special permission would be required to take it on board flights). I also gave Andrew a shave; which brought my baby back.

Tuesday and Wednesday weren't that fabulous as Andrew was

quite unwell with vomiting. As a result, he didn't have many feeds and we ceased all medications. Despite feeling quite dreadful, Andrew had some quality moments thanks to some close friends visiting and one of his insurance policies paying out.

Thursday 24th of July

Andrew was feeling a little better and a visit from a Union Official who made a special trip from Brisbane and Flight Centre advising that Cathay Pacific had approved our travel on a medical basis further buoyed his mood. Despite this, Andrew had only three to four feeds all day and was showing signs of being allergic to one of the medications he was taking. Not sure, but it appeared that he was becoming super sensitive to some things.

Our venturing to India was becoming more viable every day. Flights were paid for on Friday, although final confirmation that Andrew was 'allowed' to fly had not yet come through. No harm in being positive. We also sent a carry bag off to be modified to accommodate the BiPAP and battery for travel.

Apparently, Andrew's case had been flagged by Queensland Health for certain medications and this was discussed with Andrew's Doctor and the DON, who was also a great support to us. We also had a visit from one of the Palliative Care Nurses and the prospect of Andrew attending the Rockhampton Hospital for assessment (at Palliative Care) on return from India was discussed again. As it would save a trip back down the mountain, it would more than likely eventuate.

We waited and waited and waited, but there was still no word from Cathay Pacific on Saturday re the engineers' decision of approval for Andrew to fly. Permission had been granted on medical grounds, but the issue of Andrew's machines was still undecided. Again, the unknown! We continued planning for the trip, regardless.

Andrew had a sub-cut infusion inserted to allow him to have certain medications without having to have needles all the time. It did sting though — ouch, but Andrew didn't complain! Due to his condition, and in consultation with his Doctor, Andrew's Fentanyl patch was increased. It was also noted that when he had Pethidine, the difference in his drive to breathe was significant and he was able to stay off the machine for extended periods of time without distress or his upper body becoming red and blotchy from a lack of oxygen.

We had quite a busy afternoon with visitors, phone calls, me wielding the razor for a much-needed shave and Sue coming back to the fold (allowing Rel to go home for a bit). During Andrew's nightly routine, we discovered that he had 'hot spots' around his shoulders — certain areas were literally hot to touch. It was odd.

Despite not having confirmation re flight approval, Sunday saw us start packing for India. Not sure how, but we were going regardless of confirmation! We were approaching it like a military operation, as precision was required in relation to everything. Merle was a little worried we weren't taking enough food for Andrew, despite us having nearly a suitcase full.

While we were all a little excited that things were finally happening, we had an enormous dose of apprehension too. It was quite a busy day with a number of people dropping in to see Andrew and much to my delight, he ventured out to the lounge room. He'd not been up for a few days and he handled it really well, not feeling too sore afterwards from the lifting and moving around.

We also had some extra excitement as Lainy rode her bike for the first time without training wheels. We opened the blinds in the bedroom so Andrew could see her — a very proud moment. Proud, but bittersweet; Andrew would have loved to be the one running beside her instead of Gav. It was a very funny moment too and gave us all a giggle as Lainy was riding downhill and Gav had to give chase because she couldn't stop!

Monday 28th of July

All day, we waited and waited to hear news re Cathay Pacific's decision. It felt like I was harassing the travel agent as I called quite a few times. In the interim, Andrew had an okay day. He had lots of drinks (orally), a number of feeds and escaped the shower that we had planned. Andrew required further scripted medication so I collected the script from the hospital, drove to the Rockhampton roundabout where I met Tony and passed it on for him to have it filled. It was all a bit surreal and Tony and I joked that we were doing a 'drug run'.

The Dietician made contact and expressed concern re Andrew's food intake, or lack thereof. She wrote out a script for an alternative food source, the same volume, but increased kilo-joules. The M.N.D. Nurse also contacted to see how Andrew was travelling and to see what our plans were regarding India.

After being on tender hooks all day, Flight Centre finally called at 5pm with crushing news. Cathay Pacific had said NO. We were all totally shattered and deflated. The feeling after the call was not a happy one, but we weren't giving up. Tomorrow we would start again. We couldn't afford not to.

While we were supposed to be jetting off to India on Tuesday 29th of July, we were instead filling out more forms for different airlines. The Travel Agent's assistance was invaluable in connecting us with alternate airlines and providing support. Everyone was subdued and upset that we were still around and Andrew especially was quite withdrawn and quiet.

To further exacerbate the situation, Andrew had a shower after going to the bathroom and it left him absolutely drained and exhausted. He was totally spent, to the extent that he was hardly able to hold himself up in the chair. This made him more upset and agitated.

Amidst all this, Noah was having some tests at the Rockhampton Hospital for a health issue (which thankfully turned out to be nothing serious) and the Real Estate was showing our property at Glendale to prospective buyers.

The following day we had friends visit; one of whom rode up on their pushbike from Rockhampton. We were in awe. Their visit came at a good time as it provided a much-needed reprieve from the oppressive atmosphere, residual of Cathay Pacific's rejection. Sue, Thorlene and I went to Rocky via the hospital to have the new medical forms signed by Andrew's Doctor. We dropped the forms into the Travel Agent and the waiting game began again as she shopped around for other airlines. On our return, Rel advised that Andrew had been quite disconsolate, again highlighting the blow caused by Cathay Pacific and their rebuff.

In anticipation of some airline providing us passage to India, I planned on a treasure trove for Hudson and Lainy for the time that Andrew and I would be away. As we would both be absent and for an extended period of time (we'd only ever been away together once previously and that was when we went to Brisbane for the horror week when Andrew was diagnosed), I wrapped gifts for each of them — one for each day that we would be gone. Some were small, others large and they consisted of an array of things from clothes to lollipops and Lego to lipstick. It was just something special for the kids so when they chose a present for the day, it was a time they could think of us and no doubt they would have a smile on their faces — if only for a short while. It was also a gentle way of letting them know how long we'd be gone. As the number of presents decreased, so did the days until our return.

Fan came up on Thursday morning and unfortunately, Andrew was having a very bad day. He was getting extremely frustrated with us as we couldn't understand some of the things that he was trying to say. There was no mistaking what he was saying with his eyes though. For that, he had a real talent! He was feeling nauseas for most of the day due to excess wind building up. To help alleviate it, we purged the P.E.G. and the practice appeared to work well as it eased his discomfort and allowed him to remain on the mask.

The day did bring forth some much-needed joy, as our Travel Agent called to advise that QANTAS and Virgin Airlines were allowing us to fly! However, ecstasy was closely followed by trepidation. Had we made the right decision to go to India? Should we be going and giving it a shot or should we stay and enjoy each other while we could? Were we being selfish? Was I being selfish? The trouble with all these questions was the fact that nobody had the answers for them. Thus, you make the choice with what information you have at the time and at that time we believed (and hoped) that we were making the correct decision — for Andrew, for us and for our fledgling family.

Everything was happening all at once. We were packing like crazy and planning our trip to the nth degree; Tan and the kids came for a visit on Sunday and it was somewhat like a double celebration as it was also Tan's birthday the following day. Fan left, Sue returned, the doctor visited, we continued Andrew's physio and likely pushed to the limit as we knew that he had to become accustomed to being uncomfortable. While he too was aware of this, it didn't alter the fact that he was unimpressed with the change in the routine and he ensured that we knew his thoughts on it.

Monday 4th of August; Tan's birthday

After waiting for so long for something to happen, when it does, the anxiety that precedes it is almost unbearable. Monday was torturous. We packed within an inch of our lives — three big ports; Andrew's food, pillows, medications and clothes had precedence and our clothes and stuff was secondary. Not the type of overseas trip I had once envisioned, but you go with what you've got! Apart from our three (heavy) suitcases, we had the 'Meds Bag' (containing essential medication for travel), the two Resmed machines and the 'Sucker Bag', which was ridiculously heavy given its contents. In addition to all of this, we had a backpack filled with 'essentials' — things that may be necessary during our travel.

Amongst all the packing, we contacted the company re Andrew's bed and made arrangements for it to be serviced and fixed during the time that we were away. Travel insurance was finalised and we registered with the Australian Embassy, just to be on the safe side. There was a steady procession of visitors and well-wishing phone calls — some people are just sincere and it was nice to have the extra support. We were also able to whip Andrew through the shower and wash and cut his hair — it's amazing what excitement and anticipation can do — or it may have been attributed to his Pethidine intake!

As expected, Hudson and Lainy became quite upset and teary around bedtime, especially when they were in saying goodnight to Andrew. I stayed in with them and they settled after a while. They perked up a little when I explained about their little present caper — a present a day while mum and dad are away. Not surprisingly, they quite liked the concept. Hudson melted my heart; he said he couldn't close his eyes because I was too beautiful to look at. He also asked me where he should look to find wishing stars. What can you say to that? Children are so precious.

The house was full and people didn't leave until late and despite being very tired, sleep didn't come very easily. Despite having to get up super early, Sue and I didn't go to bed until the wee hours. The anxiety and constant thoughts about the trip, leaving the kids and all that could possibly happen were not sleep-friendly; not for any of us, but most especially for Andrew. He was putting on a brave front, but his nerves would have been the tautest of all.

India, Take Two

Tuesday 5th of August

Our journey began at 4:30am as Sue gave Andrew some anti-nausea medication. Rel and Gav arrived around 6:30am and we made final preparations, completed last minute packing, readied Andrew and I somehow changed the combination lock on one of the suitcases and didn't know the new one! Miraculously, after some fiddling, I stumbled across the new code — phew!

As our leaving time encroached, the house continued to fill up with people who came to see us off. The kids' getting-ready-for-school-routine was a little askew due to the busyness of the morning. Lainy was scheduled to have school photos taken and as the usual departing time for her to get to school on time was 7:30am, she was the first to leave. While there weren't too many theatrics, it was very hard and sad and we were all quite teary. As Hudson didn't have too far to go to get to school, he didn't have to leave until after we did. For some reason, the scenario of the kids' leaving us was somehow less painful than our leaving the kids'.

We had planned to be left by 8:30am and it was only a little after when we finally departed. Getting Andrew into the car was quite an effort, but he championed it. We said goodbye to those who weren't coming to the airport and it was difficult looking back up the driveway at everyone waving us off, especially Hudson, as he was quite upset.

Our trip to the airport wasn't too bad. On the actual journey, the biggest concern was wind, but Rel was able to expel it through Andrew's peg, which alleviated his discomfort somewhat. So, all things considered, apart from the difficulty in getting in and out of the car (as it was necessary for Andrew to be lifted and trying to keep the machine hoses from being a hindrance was tricky), the initial part of the trip was relatively good.

We had quite the little entourage at the airport with both of our Mums, Fan and Jock, Wayne and the boys, Tony and the girls and some of our friends from Blackwater. While we had our own wheelchair, it's policy for Andrew to travel on one provided by the airline. Regarding this, we waited until the very last to transfer Andrew so he'd be comfortable for as long as possible. Once through security, we didn't really have to wait that long as we were the first to board — first on last off. One thing was for sure, it was much better this time around as I was going with Andrew; not waving goodbye from the terminal.

The trek from Rocky to Brisbane wasn't a fabulous flight due to there being very little room. To top it all off, there was a short delay in leaving and when we arrived, we had the Granny of all taxi drivers, although she was a lovely lady. Being ultra-organised, we had booked the taxi in advance, but we had to walk over three zebra crossings to get to it! We figured it was about a kilometre — it definitely was not a door-to-door service!

On arrival at the International Airport, some friends and family were waiting for us. Gav, Sue and Rel took Andrew into one of the toilets to get him ready for the next flight. We didn't really have much time and once we had made it through customs, they were making the final call for our flight — Brisbane to Singapore! We absolutely legged it, giving Andrew one hell of a ride in the process.

Gav and Andrew were travelling business class and it was great as there was heaps of room and Andrew was quite comfortable as he could stretch out. Economy section — not so much. Rel went up and back a few times to see how Andrew was travelling and I had a few visits. Andrew was all set up. A lovely man sitting next to Andrew talked with the cabin crew re Andrew's circumstances and next thing we knew, we were all invited up to business class for the remainder of the trip! Wow. We couldn't believe it — the airline staff were lovely and couldn't do enough for us. Andrew seemed to be tolerating the travel — he was having Midazolam (which made him sleep), had quite a bit to drink, was moving quite a lot in the seat to try and get comfortable and he had wind. We found that the level of wind increased substantially on take-off and landing and as a result, Gav just allowed Andrew's peg to vent throughout both. It sounded like an orchestra at times!

It was quite an effort to get Andrew in and out of the plane seats due to the lifting and the lack of space made things more awkward for everyone. I'm sure it didn't look particularly coordinated, but it was, as we had to make the transition as quickly and smoothly as possible. Andrew remained the trooper and never complained — about anything.

When we arrived at Singapore, the crew and airport staff continued to be enormously supportive, to the point that they wanted to do it all. They wanted to lift Andrew onto his wheelchair, hold his machine bag, push the wheelchair and remove all of our bags from the plane. In the end, we needed to be quite firm about our independence. However, as there were so many people about and so much was happening in a very short space of time and we were watching everyone else as well as concentrating on what we needed to be doing, things were overlooked.

We were half way through the terminal when we realised the Sucker Bag was missing! Just as we realised its absence, one of the staff members accompanying us received a call on his radio advising him of same. He wasted absolutely no time and ran off to retrieve it for us, leaving us lolling about in the walkway. He then lead and settled us in a lounge area, which involved a transfer between terminals via air train! Prior to leaving us, he pre-arranged for a co-worker to pick us up and take us to our gate closer to our flight time. In the interim (which wasn't very long), we got Andrew as comfortable as we could and changed his mask and the machines.

It was all quite surreal, especially when surrounded by the hustle and bustle of the airport and the plentiful duty free shops, all of which we ignored. Everything and anything was on offer, but due to the limited time factor, we needed to be focused on Andrew and shopping was just irrelevant to our purpose (never thought that would be possible for me, but nonetheless true in this instance).

Once we arrived at the gate to check in for the flight between Singapore and Delhi, Jet Airways advised us that they had no data regarding us. We provided them with the medical forms that we had and even though we said we needed the documentation returned, he took them, showed them to the Captain and in all the hubbub and movement, we didn't realise he hadn't returned them until we were seated on the plane! And hubbub there was! We were made to give up our opened water bottles and the airline had an issue with our taking the sucker on board. Just prior to entering the plane, we had cause to utilise the sucker on Andrew and while we attempted to be discreet, it was difficult and the space didn't allow for much privacy (and we had to get the water bottles back that we had just relinquished). Following this episode, there was no issue with our taking the sucker with us.

As we were the first to board the plane, when the other passengers came on the majority of them stared, stared and stared! We attributed it to possibly being a cultural thing and our little travel party was obviously not something people are exposed to every day, but in some instances, people's behaviour was just plain rude and inexcusable. There was a small majority of passengers who gave kind wishes and get-well comments.

Again, Gav and Andrew were seated in business class and Rel may as well have been as she spent most of the flight up there. Sue and I were down the back in the throng! However, we did eat and sleep quite a bit throughout the flight and on one of Rel's trips back to see us, she said we were both lights out with our dinner trays on our laps.

This leg of the trip wasn't particularly good for Andrew as his chair wasn't as comfortable and there wasn't a lot of room. Besides that, Andrew's machine kept going off (beeping), which it tended to do if the seal of the mask was compromised. (Sometimes, if Andrew slept or moved his face in a certain way, the seal of the mask was broken and the machine would beep to alert of this.)

From stories told after the first trip to India, Sue and I weren't expecting much when we arrived at the airport in Delhi. We were very pleasantly surprised to find that not only did they have a chair lift to unload us, we entered a sparkly new flash terminal — nothing resembling the terminal our lot remembered from their previous visit. Andrew, Rel and Gav were all shocked by the transformation. The new terminal had only been opened a matter of months so they must have started operations just after they left the last time.

We whizzed through customs and I was a little annoyed as I'd left my Fantales on the plane, thinking they wouldn't be allowed in as the packet was opened and they were dairy. They didn't even check!

We were very well looked after within the terminal. The airport staff pushed Andrew's chair (under our close supervision) and they sought out our escort. We were impressed with the service we received, but saddened by the beggars outside the terminal. After the journey, we had endured though, Andrew was absolutely done. It was a nice surprise, and somewhat of a comfort, to see that the same guy that had collected them on their initial visit was there again and they had both a car and an ambulance waiting for us.

We weren't really bothered by the people outside the terminal, but there was one guy who kept opening Gav's door and asking for stuff. We initially thought he was with the hospital staff, but he wasn't and Gav pretty much told him to 'go away'. In the end, it was decided that Gav would go with Andrew in the ambulance and their protocols saw Andrew transferred to a stretcher for the trip to the hospital. After we all pulled away from the airport, we realised that we hadn't given Gav another machine for Andrew — just in case. We pretty much had all the excess gear with us and while it wasn't required, it scared the bejesus out of us knowing that if they did need it, they wouldn't have had it!

The car trip to the hospital was... different. It was 3am, drizzly and quite manic. We figured the traffic must be absolute murder at peak hour. The stories that the guys relayed to us about 'no rules' were quite true and only some people recognised the traffic lights. Horns blared all over the place, despite the early hour and believe me, it was an experience. There was an uncanny amount of action happening even though it was the very early hours of the morning.

After leaving the mainstream traffic and going through what seemed like back alleys and such for quite a while, we arrived at a gate, which happened to be locked. Meanwhile, we had lost visual contact with the ambulance and had no idea of where our boys were — this was a terrifying prospect, as we had no conceivable way of contacting them or knowing how they were doing. We took another route and soon were at the hospital. After a short wait, the ambulance arrived with Andrew and Gav. The relief of seeing them was immeasurable. We were all incredibly tired, but we helped the staff unload Andrew from the ambulance and get him into the hospital. This was easier said than done as the gradient of their ramp was significant and there were a few of us standing and assisting from behind, as it was very steep.

We were assigned one of the 'post-operative' rooms and while it was quite basic, it was spacious and had air conditioning. As his entourage, we were provided with a room one floor up at the hospital, but we decided at the first instance that we were all going to stay together, no matter what; A slumber party of sorts. What was going to happen was going to happen with us all present and accounted for. While we were all ridiculously tired, it applied to Andrew tenfold, but despite our fatigue, we were all elated to have finally arrived and get the next stage started. We had made it and that, in and of itself, was an achievement.

Day 1 in India — Wednesday 6th of August

We were all pretty shattered and slept on and off all day. Being so tall, Andrew didn't quite fit in the hospital bed, so we had to put his feet out through the railings at the bottom. Not ideal, or that comfortable, but he did manage to see the humour in the situation. Doctor S. visited us fairly early and she appeared quite happy with Andrew and his condition. She maintained that he's too young for M.N.D. and wasn't convinced that this was what ailed him. She was very positive and upbeat and it was difficult not to draw strength from her and have hope. If nothing else, she was a champion invigorator and instiller of hope.

Doctor S. had arranged a room for us at her clinic (as opposed to the Hospital) as she wanted us to be looked after as well as Andrew. She felt that we all needed to be as well as we could be to care for Andrew and to do this, we needed to be looked after ourselves. Her philosophy envisioned us receiving sufficient rest, which would assist in optimising the results.

Leaving Gav with Andrew, Rel, Sue and I ventured over to the clinic to have a shower and general freshen up. Wow! Things were really different over here. The traffic was extremely chaotic, but somehow it seemed to work. The constant blaring of horns was somehow orchestrated to how it all progressed, surprisingly, without incident. We were startled by the traffic on the roads and what it actually entailed — everything from people, animals (of all shapes and sizes), bikes, scooters, motorbikes (sometimes with up to three or four passengers), buses, wagons, tut-tuts, cars, trucks — you name it, it was on the road!

There were sights everywhere. One didn't know where to look. There were people like you had never seen before, washing was hanging off anything and everything, cows were wandering everywhere — even in the middle of traffic — there were no lines of traffic to speak of, but there was some order within the chaos as there was consistent horn blaring and what appeared to be few incidents or accidents. Motorbikes whizzed in and out and tried to make it through the smallest of cracks in traffic, people were actually living on the street — a family under some stairs, one under an umbrella and cardboard, others under a set of trees and they were cooking on the sidewalk. A reality check, if nothing else.

The Clinic was situated on a very busy street and one of the neighbouring buildings housed a bank and it was complete with armed guards — scary! The Clinic itself was significantly more modern than the Hospital and unlike the latter, we didn't have to take our shoes off to go into the rooms and put on the thongs provided. Our first visit was inspirational due to the people we met whilst there. One girl, who happened to hail from Australia, had suffered a spinal injury and had been there for a months' treatment. She was hoping to stay until the end of the year as she had quantified amazing results in the short time she'd been there.

On our return to the hospital, in a tut-tut, we went through various markets and shop fronts. Everything was colourful, busy and frenzied. Much to my dismay, we went past the 'chicken shop', but I didn't see it. Given the reports from their last visit, this shop was definitely on the 'to see' list!

The physiotherapist came and assessed Andrew and one of the doctors came in during the afternoon for his first session of physio. She was scheduled to visit daily at 1:40pm. Following the session, Andrew was absolutely shattered and he slept for quite a while. Apart from trying to lie on his sides more, which he found quite comfortable for short periods, Andrew was also encouraged to breathe through his nose more.

We considered ourselves to be very fortunate as we had a TV. Animal Planet and the National Geographic channels were the stations of choice. The sitcoms and other shows were not as interesting or funny in Indian.

We had some difficulty fitting the adapters into the power sockets and we had to call on some of the hospital staff to assist us. The system was quite antiquated and it was frightening to see that even the guys that helped us had trouble plugging things in. At one stage, one of them used pens and pliers to plug some of the things in. It was terrifying to watch, especially when you could see the sparks and hear the crackle of the electricity. We were supplied with three power boards, which we found easier to utilise. We had a few heart-stopping moments when all of the batteries for Andrew's machine were running low and we couldn't plug things in! With help, we soon had them charging, although the whole time we were using their power, we were afraid the electricity would fail or surge. We were assured there were backup generators for the hospital should there be a power outage, but regardless of this, we tried to make sure we charged the batteries as often as possible.

Andrew wasn't overly comfortable in the hospital bed — not surprising considering, a) he was used to his 'you beaut' bed at home and, b) he was too big for it. We advised the staff and in an effort to make it more restful for him, they plan to bring an air mattress tomorrow. They would have brought it today, but Andrew was too tired to get up for it to go on the bed.

The cells started today! Andrew had three lots throughout the day, some I.M. and some I.V. It was quite incredible to see Andrew actually getting the treatment. It's what we travelled around the world for. There was so much riding on those injections; hard to believe all of our hopes rested on them. Andrew also started on another course of antibiotics.

We had doctors, nurses and other hospital staff coming and going all day. They were all extremely nice and couldn't do enough for us. It was like Grand Central Station. While we had the room at the clinic, we all decided that we didn't want to be separated so we would all bunk in the ol' operating theatre together. It was like a slumber party that had no end time.

We called home and I talked with mum and the kids. It was good to hear their voices, but a little sad too. I assured them I was madly clicking away with the camera so they could see India as we were and there were many sights to behold — some amazing, some baffling and some were just seeing-is-believing. The kids were also ultra-excited about the whole present-a-day deal and couldn't wait for their next instalment.

Day 2 — Thursday 7th of August

Even though we'd only been there for a very short time, so much had happened and it literally felt like we'd been there for ages. Doctor S. visited early and we discussed Andrew's case. She was of the belief that Andrew's food (via the P.E.G.) was for maintenance purposes only and that he required good, real nutrition. She had given the kitchen orders to send up meals that could be vitamised twice daily and in having it, he would be provided with all he required. On trying it, Andrew felt very uncomfortable, but that was more because he wasn't used to having 'real' food, per say.

Doctor S. also focused on Andrew's breathing and encouraged him to breathe for himself, even when he's on the machine. While the machine does it for him, she expressed concern that his muscles weren't working at all and his allowing the machine to breathe for him was a habit. Besides that, the cells wouldn't know that there was anything wrong if Andrew didn't use his muscles to breathe. In allowing the machine to do it all, the cells would think things were progressing normally and they would have no reason to target Andrew's respiratory system and this certainly was not the case. The rate of breathing was also an issue of contention as she felt it was set too high. This, in turn, encouraged Andrew not to breathe himself, as it would prove to be too exhausting over prolonged periods of time.

Physiotherapy was scheduled for twice-daily visits — once in the morning to focus on Andrew's chest area for breathing and the other in the afternoon, which concentrated on the rest of his body. Andrew felt very tired, but quite good following his sessions, especially in the shoulder region. He felt he had more movement and with that, he shrugged his shoulders! It was a huge improvement and we were mightily impressed. It was great to see Andrew being so positive, even though it was obvious that he was tired and in pain.

Doctor A. came and gave Andrew his stem cell injection intercostally; between the ribs. It was painful to watch and seemed quite tricky (that's why Doctor A. was doing it), but it was a necessary part of the process so Andrew received it as thought it was an everyday occurrence — someone sticking needles in between his ribs.

Andrew was also happy and felt a huge difference after an airbed was placed on top of his mattress. His comfort level had been quite okay and was not as big an issue as we had anticipated it being. Not yet, anyway.

Right outside the hospital was a park and play area and on one of my visits beyond the operating room, I encountered my first squirrel. I was taking heaps of pictures of the squirrel, my surroundings and the local children when a lady approached me and led me to her home (it was within very close proximity to the hospital). While we were unable to communicate through words, she wanted me to take pictures of her and her family. I complied and she was extremely friendly and most thankful.

Gav and I took a trip back to the clinic to gather supplies. The chaos of the traffic was still quite unbelievable, but it flowed none-the-less and the horns blaring were all a part of the whole scenario. We travelled via tut-tut, which somehow added authenticity and interest to the experience. We followed the same route as the day before and as such, I was prepared with the camera when we passed the people on the street working with the flowers and the chicken shop!

Made contact with Flight Centre and requested that medical forms for QANTAS and Jet Airways be forwarded to us (for the return journey). While they may not have been required, we thought it better to be thorough and safe-than-sorry.

Andrew felt quite unwell and was uncomfortable for the majority of the afternoon and we put a lot of it down to his not being used to tolerating the heaviness of the food he was having. To counter this, we planned to water the food down more and introduce it at a slower rate.

There were a few domestic issues that we had to work through. They provided us with thimble-sized cups, which didn't make for very satisfying cups of tea and hot, not boiling water for said cups of tea. We also sourced a bucket to do our own washing up. Sue likened it to camping!

Day 3 — Friday 8th of August

Throughout the course of the day, Andrew received five lots of cells — two x I.M., one x I.V. infusion and two x intercostal.

Andrew was due to have an ultra-sound around 8:30am so we plied him with lots of water in anticipation. Unfortunately, the test was postponed for an hour so he was tremendously uncomfortable and bloated. The ultra-sound showed that Andrew had a small kidney stone on the left, but due to its size, nothing specific needed to be done, apart from keeping him well hydrated.

We chatted with one of the nurses assigned to Andrew. She was from north-east India and had been at the hospital for about two years. We discovered that training and working conditions are certainly different to what we were used to.

Sue was very busy organising, packing and moving things around. We teased her about taking over 'Sharon's' position. He was the domestic assigned to us. He came in every day, sometimes a few times a day. He was always friendly and despite the language barrier, we communicated quite well.

A shower chair was brought over from the clinic to make it easier for Andrew to use the rooms' facilities. It was good timing and we didn't waste any in using it. True to form though, the experience was not without drama as the chair broke. Regrettably, Andrew was on it at the time! The seat came off and the wheels of the chair wouldn't turn. As we were in the bathroom, there was very little room for us to help Andrew and it was quite a precarious position for him to be in. The entire venture was not overly successful and Andrew was quite upset. We all were. Once the ordeal was over, we unanimously concurred that we would have to devise another plan for the future, as the shower chair was no longer an option.

On top of everything else, we alternated masks every six hours or so as the skin on Andrew's nose had been compromised and needed to be rested.

The kitchen sent up chicken soup that we vitamised for Andrew. We added resource, but having learnt from yesterday, only gave him very small amounts at the one time. We were also adding resource to Andrew's Fortisip meals to increase his intake.

Rel, Sue and I went to 'the shops' via tut-tut. The driver we had didn't seem to have any idea of where to go (and this may have been due to the language barrier), but we eventually made it. It took a while to get there, but we didn't mind overly much as we considered it an extra sightseeing opportunity. I thought we were at the markets, but it ended up being the higher-end shops. Each shop had a different footpath and it was extremely uneven (would have been a killer in heels). To make the experience more interesting, it was raining and it was heartbreakingly sad when a little boy approached us and was asking for money.

I was surprised that most of the shops' wares were similar to what one may find at home — such as Barbie and Transformers. We didn't spend a lot of time, but we brought Andrew a squeeze ball, four decent sized coffee cups, some Pringles and a washing up dish and detergent.

There didn't appear to be a dull moment as on the way back to the hospital, our tut-tut nearly disappeared down a hole in the road! We saw a lot of cows just roaming around and I actually saw the chicken man sitting up on his block in the shop! Sue missed it because my head was in the way, so we vowed to go back at a later date.

We had phone calls back home and talked with some of the staff about India and Australia. Andrew did various exercises throughout the day, although he didn't have physio (as such) because the doctor didn't arrive. Regardless, he was absolutely shattered and had to have something to help him settle.

Day 4 — Saturday 9th of August

Andrew had three lots of cells today — two x I.M. and one x I.V. infusion.

It's been established that I am not a good candidate for the night shift and I am able to sleep quite soundly. This was proven as Andrew's machine continually went off during the night (due to his mask leaking) and the other guys had to use the sucker (which is ridiculously loud) and I slept on oblivious. Poor Andrew and the others didn't get much sleep at all.

Sue and I are both feeling a little off — a touch fluey, so we are taking every precaution.

Merle called very early to let us know that Hudson won the colouring competition at the Mount Morgan Show. Wow!! Mum also sent photos of the kids at soccer and they are excited to be going off to the Mount Morgan Show later today. In contrast, we didn't venture out at all. We lazed about, reading, snoozing, watching the Olympic highlights (most of which referred to the Indian athletes) and playing cards.

Andrew had another physiotherapist visit and they did a few different things. We also gave him the stress ball we purchased yesterday and he used it with both hands, although I assisted him with his right. On the whole, he says he doesn't really feel any different, and it's unknown if it's related or not, but when Andrew's off the machine, he's not going red at all. Is it the cells? Is it the vitamised food he's having as well as his peg feeds? Is it our imaginations? It would be nice to have answers to these questions. It would be nice to have answers to any of our questions.

On a lighter note, the 'kissan jam' was delicious as it tasted just like raspberry pops and while I dabbled in the yumminess of it all, Andrew had his resource and milk. It's a bit of a reality check. Hailing from the Mount, it was not surprising that we were constantly requesting boiling water from the kitchen (for our cups of tea). However, we were assured that this was not an imposition as they had hired an extra person for the kitchen.

Shying away from a full-blown shower, we gave Andrew a wash. His ribs were quite sore and he had quite a few bruises coming out as a result of our last efforts.

Day 5 — Sunday 10th of August

Andrew had three lots of cells today — two x I.M. and one x I.V. infusion.

I was a little excited as I nearly did a night shift! I stayed up until 3am before succumbing to sleep. I slept long and hard afterwards though.

We had a very lazy day and while we contemplated going back to the clinic, it didn't eventuate. Andrew watched a movie on the iPod that friends had given him for the trip. We watched telly, which was more exciting, as we found a channel showing the Olympics. Andrew had his physio, I then rang and talked to the kids and we played cards.

Andrew wasn't having feeds as regularly as we would have liked, but he indicated that he was feeling bloated/ full most of the time. Sue and I were probably guilty of bullying him into having feeds sometimes, but it was all for the greater good... we hoped.

Day 6 — Monday 11th of August

Andrew had three lots of cells today — one x I.M. and two x I.V. infusion. Doctor S. informed that she was using a new formula/ concoction and she was supplying Andrew with massive (larger than normal) doses.

WOW! Things were really happening. I woke up and the first thing I saw was Andrew moving his right hand! He was wiggling his fingers, shrugging his shoulders and moving his arms! To put it mildly, we were gob-smacked, especially considering that Andrew hadn't had a lot of movement in his right hand for about three months! Considering he could barely hold a ball in his hand a mere two days ago, the new movement was astonishing to say the least!

Not long after the mornings' excitement, Doctor S. arrived and on hearing of Andrew's improvements, she expressed her desire for Andrew to stay longer. She arranged for Andrew to have a HUGE dose of cells (I.V.) — twice as many cells as last time. She also requested that he sit on the side of the bed with his legs hanging over the edge and he continue with his breathing and movement exercises.

We made attempts to call 'The Mums' with our exciting news, but they were at bingo! Ha, Ha. After Andrew had rested for a while, we videoed his progress and sent the footage home via phone and the response we received was very positive and energising. Merle's reaction was especially priceless (once she returned home from bingo) and highlighted why we were half way across the world doing what we were doing — for hope.

Despite the triumphs of the day, we still had to continue monitoring other elements of Andrew's condition, such as his oxygen saturation levels and food intake. Just because we seemingly had a breakthrough in one area, we couldn't be blasé and ignore everything else.

Not sure if it was from the stress of all that was occurring or just my intrinsic make-up, but I needed to shop. I was actually dreaming about it (I am obviously one who uses this as a method of stress relief — no surprises there!) and we talked to a couple of the nurses about options that we had. We had a bathroom visit that, thankfully, was much more successful than the last episode and following that, Rel, Sue and I returned to the Clinic to have a break and freshen up.

On our way there, we indulged in some retail therapy by visiting the shops at Green Park. We went into a sweet shop and it was literally a child's dream shop. It was otherworldly and transportive and I loved it! We tumbled back to Earth, however, when we returned to our designated unit at The Clinic. Imagine our surprise when we discovered that the shower roof had collapsed! We called maintenance and they cleaned things up pronto and even though we were hoping the incident had not been our fault, we tried not to think about it and enjoyed our shower regardless.

On leaving The Clinic, we tried to return the key as we were all staying at the old hospital, but they refused to accept it. Instead of arguing the point, we simply returned the key at a later time, reiterating that we did not need it, as we were all happy to share the room at the hospital.

In all my wisdom, I didn't pack the battery charger for the camera and sure enough — the battery was going flat; lightning fast! Not surprising really, when you consider I was clicking away at everything and anything. Hmmm. Where to get another battery? If one wasn't available, do I buy another camera altogether? Questions, questions, questions!

We continued to have a few communication issues with the domestic staff at the hospital. On this occasion, we requested more towels, but the message was difficult to get across. We ended up having to say, "You know, the things you dry yourself with after a shower?" We eventually received the extra towels and the episode left us giggling.

All in all, today was a good day. It was long and a lot happened. Despite the power outages (and thank goodness for the batteries) it was exciting, gratifying, but best of all Andrew had the spark back in his eyes. He was feeling better within himself, stronger, more balanced and hope was renewed.

Day 7 — Tuesday 12th of August

Andrew had five lots of cells today — two x I.M. and three x I.V. One of the latter was a bigger than normal dose.

Had a visit from Doctor S, who was happy with the improvement of Andrew's condition. His ability to move was increasing and he felt stronger and while this was fantastic, he was doing so much moving by himself that he was tiring himself out. That was Andrew, through and through. Going above and beyond the physio sessions, he was extending himself to the point of exhaustion!

Gav and I approached Doctor S re Andrew's treatment, both here and on our return to Australia, his drug requirements (antibiotics, pain medications and such), her visiting Australia in October and payment. She provided scripts for the medications Andrew needed (three months' supply — she also advised that such medications were a lot cheaper in India than Australia and the point was taken!). With regards to payment, she informed us that there was nothing owing for the current treatment Andrew was receiving, as there were still monies left from the initial payment we made prior to the first pilgrimage. Wow! We certainly weren't expecting that, but it was welcomed.

Sue, Rel and I journeyed to the S.N. Markets and we decided it was nothing like the Calliope Markets at home. There were hordes of hawkers and beggars who incessantly approached us with their wares or simply asked for money. The majority of beggars were young children and while our hearts melted with sadness, we steeled ourselves against their pleas. If we had relented, we would have been swamped, as there were so many of them — we couldn't help them all.

Amazingly, I was able to find a battery charger for the camera. Go Kodak! Even more unbelievable was how inexpensive it was. So too were the other bits and pieces we purchased — an authentic

Indian sari, an outfit for Lainy, shoes (no shopping expedition is complete without them), watches and sunglasses. We were fortunate in the sense that we didn't need to utilise the public bathroom facilities as they were open-air and the temptation of refreshments were countered by the obvious lack of food safety regulations. The lemonade stand was certainly an eye opener!

On our return to the hospital, Gav said they had had a visit from a lady whose husband also had M.N.D. She and her husband had relocated their family (they have two children, 8 and 11) from Brisbane to New Delhi so he could receive on-going treatment. They too sought treatment 'outside the box' because they weren't satisfied with the advice they received in Australia.

Talked with Mum and was happy to hear about the excitement Andrew's movements incited and that the kids were doing great. I thought about them even more after learning of the above lady's story and mirroring our situation with theirs. I don't know that I'd have the courage to move the entire family on a permanent basis, especially not so far away from support and to a foreign country. Her strength, bravery and optimism was uplifting, to say the least, and knowing we weren't the only ones going through the M.N.D. voyage was a comfort, of sorts.

Mum also advised that there was a guy travelling up from Brisbane to repair Andrew's bed. We relayed the issues regarding the bed to Dad, as he would be our go-between.

The importance of feeding Andrew (and the cells) 'real' food was not always met with enthusiasm as he was often reluctant to have things orally. In support of this reluctance, after having some chicken broth, Andrew's throat became tickly and he was not happy, especially because the discomfort lasted a few hours. We were treated to whole fish for our dinner. They looked like piranhas, but they didn't taste too bad and there was no curry so we didn't complain too much.

Day 8 – Wednesday 13th of August

Andrew had seven lots of cells today — two x I.M., two x I.V. (one big needle), two x intercostal and one x spine/neck

We were all up quite early, as Andrew wanted to have completed his exercises prior to Doctor S's visit, which he did. During her visit, Andrew actually sat on the side of the bed and was able to do so unaided for a short while. He could move his legs/muscles and indicated that it felt good just to be able to sit up. Doctor S. also had Andrew hold a pen (we purchased a small whiteboard the other day for this purpose) and we were all excited as he wrote 'AND' with his left hand! Given his progress thus far, Doctor S. encouraged Andrew to keep up with his exercises, especially his breathing and she also promoted the use of yoga and meditation. She further motivated him by saying that it was a shared goal to have him go back to Brisbane (his Doctors) and say, "Here I am!" As expected, Andrew was pretty tired after the morning's activities, but despite this, we did his morning routine, gave him a shave and then he went to the bathroom. Following this, he was absolutely whacked.

Doctor S. and Doctor A. visited again later in the day and Doctor A. administered Andrew's intercostal and spine needles. According to Andrew, the intercostal ones hurt more, but as a bystander, I wasn't convinced.

Gav, Sue and I went to the Clinic to attend a meeting between the doctors and patients. You were able to ask questions and as such, it was very informative and interesting to learn of other people's stories. We met some of the other patients and their carers' and their ailments included M.N.D. and Lime Disease, but the majority had suffered spinal injuries. It was fascinating listening to Doctor S. and her team. She advised that all of the cells used to date, for all of the patients, have originated from the one embryo. Therefore, in a sense, all that had received them have a unique connection. She further explained that improvement and/or movement within a few days of treatment is the stem cells activating the body's dormant cells, but it takes a long time to regenerate the core of the cells.

On our return trip to the hospital, we saw many funny and interesting sights. While realising that cows are considered sacred, it was quite astounding to see one asleep in the middle of a very busy road and the traffic just whizzed around it as though it was a permanent feature and was nothing out of the ordinary. We also saw a man ironing on the side of the road. He had what appeared to be a permanent board/table set up and was using an enormously large and heavy iron.

We stopped in at the Green Park shops to exchange some money so we could pay for the medications we would be purchasing in India to take home. Locating the exchange was a bit like finding a needle in a haystack, but we did get there eventually. We also went in to McDonalds to get some rupee change. It smelled a little like the McDonalds at home, but we figured fries are fries, no matter where you are. As Gav had the money, Sue and I asked him to get us an ice-cream, as we wanted to see whether it tasted the same. To our amusement, he said no because he didn't think we'd have enough rupee to get us back to the hospital. It was hilarious. We felt a little like naughty kids and we didn't let him live it down!

Andrew continued with his exercises, using the squeeze ball, holding a pen and doing some writing with his left hand. While being in the very early stages of treatment and its positive effects, we were all feeling great as it seemed we had made a little u turn on our highway to hell! We were all hoping our direction remained on this course and it wasn't just a detour.

Pizza was delivered for tea and the kitchen sent us some rice dishes as well. After nearly polishing off all of my rice, I found something foreign in it and while I didn't know what it was, it was hairy and succeeded in souring my appetite for Indian cuisine! Andrew especially thought the episode very funny. Me; not so much!

Day 9 — Thursday 14th of August

Andrew had six lots of cells today — two x I.M., one x I.V. (large dose), two x intercostal and one x spine/neck

Doctor S. visited early again and she shared information concerning another of her M.N.D. patients. They had been receiving treatment for longer than Andrew, were doing extremely well and were regaining abilities that the disease had rid them of. She also advised that paperwork from the airlines (requiring her attention as Andrew's Doctor) had not yet come through. Given that tomorrow was a public holiday in India for their Independence Day, it needed to come through today. Regarding this, we attempted to make contact with Flight Centre and when this wasn't successful, Thorlene made enquiries on our behalf. We eventually received the paperwork via email, but due to incompatibility of programs, we couldn't understand it!

Despite the drama with the paperwork, Andrew was feeling good and looking better than he had. He was feeling especially strong in the neck area, as he was able to hold his head up for long periods. Along with letters for our travel pertaining to Andrew's health status, clearance to travel and the medications we would be travelling home with, Doctor S. gave Andrew a pep talk re he can do anything. It was very positive for all of us.

Made contact with home and Mum advised that while the kids were missing us, they were doing fine and things were continuing on for them as normal. She also reported that two guys visited and fixed Andrew's bed. It took them seven hours!

Andrew started feeling off during the course of the day. He indicated that his breathing was harder and aside from his two sessions of physio and the breathing exercises, he did little else. His back was also sore from constantly laying down.

One of the staff came to see how we were all travelling and told us there were local markets happening that night. Never ones to pass up a shopping opportunity, Sue, Rel and I braved the elements — it was storming — and checked it out. While it wasn't quite what we were expecting, it was very basic and interesting to see the realness of everyday life for these people. Restaurants were identified by large pots of food boiling out in the open, one stall sold flour out of large bags and it was doled out by a huge scoop and weighed on an over-sized set of scales and there were a few places of worship lit with candles dotted around. On the short walk to and from the market street, we passed by many homes. They consisted of rooms that were very small and sparsely furnished and many were crowded with people and had water covering the floor. It was eye opening and certainly fostered appreciation for all that we have at home.

Apart from our venture to the market, we didn't go out today. We played cards, read, Andrew watched a movie on the iPod and we watched some Animal Planet. McDonalds has a new add showing constantly on TV and their new slogan is, "I'm loving it." We definitely were not!

We are all a little over the food and as such, we had toast for tea. We also continued to experience difficulty in getting boiling water, as the kitchen would only send us hot water. It certainly didn't make for a decent cuppa!

I also noticed some weird marks/bites on my neck and they were itchy. It was freaking me out!

Day 10 — Friday 15th of August; India's Independence Day

Andrew had three lots of cells today — two x I.M., one x I.V. infusion

Sam (Helen's youngest daughter) had her baby this morning.

Unfortunately, my bites didn't disappear overnight and I showed one of the doctors when they came to see Andrew. She had some cream sent up for me from the chemist attached to the hospital.

Andrew was in quite a playful mood during his exercises. He didn't have physio, per say, due to it being Independence Day, but we did our own version. There were a few tense moments with his machines/batteries, but it was likely more to do with the connections for the power than the equipment itself. The electrical set up was quite scary with all its wiggling and sparking!

We decided not to make the trip to the Clinic for the Independence Day celebrations. Andrew certainly wasn't up to the trip as his playful mood and sense of wellbeing deteriorated as the afternoon progressed. We all stayed in and filled our time watching movies and playing cards. We did hear fireworks throughout the evening — or what we thought and hoped were fireworks!

We made contact with home and were so envious as the kids told us they went to Sizzler! We could almost taste it, especially considering we had cereal, soup and toast for dinner!

While talking with the kids and catching up on what they were up to was great, it also made me miss them more. They sounded so grown up. We were all counting down the days until we returned home and we even put in our order for our return dinner on Tuesday night — roast pork and lamb, vegetables (sans the curry!), pumpkin soup and dessert.

Day 11 – Saturday 16th of August

Andrew had four lots of cells today — two x I.M, one x I.V. infusion and one huge needle — thirty times the normal dose

First up in the morning, we organised and paid for the ambulance and taxi for our trip to the airport on Monday morning — 5:30am pick up! Gav also made an early call to the lady that had visited Andrew earlier and arranged for us to visit her and her family at their home later that day.

Andrew felt off for most of the day. He had a lot of wind and following his physio, one of his shoulders became very sore which made him very uncomfortable.

Sue stayed with Andrew and Rel, Gav and I went to the Green Park shops. We brought some souvenir gifts for everyone at home and we planned to see the chicken man on the way back to the hospital, but the tut-tut driver took a different route! Our journey back was not uneventful though, as the driver went the wrong way up the main street as a short cut and Gav saw a hole in the road that appeared to be bottomless.

Rel stayed with Andrew and Sue, Gav and I met with a driver at 4pm and he took us to the lady visitor's home, which was about twenty minutes away. Her family lived in a gated community and while things on the outside appeared closed in and crowded, the inside was quite spacious. Her husband was a little older than Andrew when diagnosed and they moved their family over to India permanently so he could receive on-going stem cell treatment. Their children attended an international school and they had live-in nursing assistance. One thing was abundantly clear to all of us from the outset and that was the courage and bravery shown by both of them. Our visit was certainly food for thought. We were treated to roast lamb for dinner and some fabulous scotch. Luckily, Sue made sure Gav and I made it back to the hospital all right!

During our absence, the Doctors visited Andrew and gave him a massive dose of cells. It was around thirty times bigger than the normal dose.

Day 12 — Sunday 17th of August

Andrew had six lots of cells today — four x I.M., one x I.V. and another massive dose — thirty times the normal dose.

It was hard to fathom that this was our last day and to top things off, it was raining. Unfortunately, this put paid to my intentions to visit the chicken man, but we were busy enough making sure we had everything packed and ready for the journey home.

I continued to be plagued by the Indian bug bites and was put on antibiotics. Apparently, such things are not uncommon during the rainy season. I just hoped they wouldn't continue to be a problem and I wouldn't be taking something sinister home with us.

Rel talked with one of the other patients at the hospital and he asked after Andrew. He advised that Doctor S. had told him, and others, about Andrew's progress. Not long after, the man's wife came up to our room and delved further into Andrew's treatment and progress.

Animal Planet made another appearance and we played some more cards. In between times, Andrew had a wash and we gave him a shave. Doctor S. visited in the early evening and during our discussion, she advised that Andrew had had more cells in the short time he had been in India, than anyone else — ever. She requested that we document all the improvements that we had noted since coming to India. From 06/08 — 18/08, we came up with:

- Overall increase of body strength;
- Return of muscle mass — legs, arms, shoulders, hands and chest;
- Return of movement to right arm and hand;
- Able to lift/shrug shoulders;
- Increased neck control and strength;
- Able to brace upper body to assist with lifting;
- Able to lift pelvis off bed;
- Increased ability to control leg movements;
- Improvement in peripheral flushing of chest when off BiPAP for period of time; and
- General increase in feeling of wellbeing.

Throughout the day, we said good-bye to the people/staff at the hospital and in our bid to be ultra-organised and not miss our flight home, we planned to retire early. That did not happen. Rel stayed up all night, I stayed up most of the night, Sue stayed up some of the night and Gav and Andrew zonked out for the whole night.

Monday morning was a very early start as we stirred around 4ish. Last minute packing was completed; machines and batteries were arranged and the process for using them on the way home was finalized; Andrew's routine was done and we were all ripe and ready when the taxi and ambulance arrived to take us to the airport. As the Hospital neighbourhood was gated and locked at the early hour of our departure, Andrew had to be wheeled out to meet the ambulance on a stretcher. It was all quite surreal, but we were ready to go home and were happy the journey had started to get us there.

The ambulance used the sirens and flashing lights all the way to the airport. Amazingly, it was also pulled over for a security check! Looking around New Delhi on our way to the airport was quite unreal. There were some beautiful sights, but there were also those that made us realise how lucky we were to just be visitors and be on our way home. Even stopping at traffic lights was an experience as we had people knocking on the windows requesting our attention and wanting us to buy things from them.

On arrival at the airport, there were guards with machine guns stationed at the entrances. It was quite off-putting, more than a little scary and we gave them a wide birth. The airport staff were very friendly and extremely helpful, but strangely enough, there were still issues with our travel. It appeared they did not have our documentation. As such, the Jet Airways doctor came and saw Andrew and asked us questions about his condition and the machines. One supervisor in particular was fantastic and she seemed to hasten proceedings for us. In the interim, she arranged for us to be seated in one of the waiting lounges and they brought up sandwiches and beverages while we waited.

Our luck didn't change going through immigration, as the person we had was painfully slow and extremely serious. Likewise, going through security. We had to take all of the machines/ batteries out of their bags and they made us take the sucker out of its bag and they then proceeded to re-check the bag through the x-ray machine. Security also had an issue with Andrew's feeds (the Fortisip) and it was necessary for us to show them the Doctor's letter re it being necessary. On finally making it to the departure lounge, Andrew needed suction and the staff continued to be very helpful. The supervisor that had assisted us earlier even came out to the plane with us, gave us hugs and wished us the best for the future.

Rel spent the majority of the flight to Singapore in business class with Andrew and Gav. Sue and I chilled and slept in the back. We also ate — of course. Prior to seating Andrew, we placed the eggshell mattress on his chair in an effort to make it more comfortable. He also required medications during the trip to further ensure his comfort.

Once we arrived in Singapore, we went off to find out where and when we needed to catch our connecting flight. From our experiences to date, this stopover was very different as we were basically left to our own devices and weren't overrun by people wanting to help. After finding out what we needed to, we ventured upstairs and went into the Qantas Lounge as it provided space and relative privacy compared to the remainder of the terminal. We moved Andrew out of the wheelchair and he laid on the lounge for a while. Our flight was delayed, but this worked in our favour as we needed the extra time to prepare Andrew for the next part of the journey.

There were some perks to Andrew being in a wheelchair, as we didn't have to join the horrendously long line-up. Instead, we were the first to board our flight, but this advantage was short-lived, as Andrew required further suctioning and attention once seated on the plane. Again, Rel spent the majority of the flight with the boys, making sure Andrew was as comfortable as he could be. We were all weary by this point, but the travelling was taking its toll on Andrew the most.

Arriving in Brisbane was sweet, although we were almost too tired to appreciate it. My Aunty Tricia met us at the airport and it was nice to see a familiar face. QANTAS endeared themselves to us further as they were aware of our desire to make the earliest connecting flight to Rockhampton and they did all they could to expedite the process. They even paid for the cab to take us to the Domestic Terminal, even though we were flying with a rival airline.

Home Again

Tuesday 19th of August

As we were able to catch the earlier flight, everything at the Domestic Terminal was rush, rush, rush. The airline staff were great and assisted us in getting to the plane on time and intact. Thankfully, the flight was very short compared to those we had just experienced and we were back in Rockhampton before 10am.

Tony, Wayne and the boys and Dad met us at the airport. Andrew was shattered and had very limited reserves left so we wasted no time in packing things up and heading home. The house was bursting with people, but the main focus was on getting Andrew into his bed so he could rest. Dad had made a disc to assist in moving Andrew from one thing to another. It made things easier and required less effort on Andrew's part, which was much appreciated. Despite what he'd been through and how he must have been feeling, Andrew championed on and gave a few demonstrations of his regained movements throughout the day.

Both the kids came home from school at lunch and we were overjoyed to see them. Lainy and Hudson were very happy to have us home and Lainy became my little shadow, which I didn't mind at all. It didn't take long to settle back in and we spent the remainder of the day talking about our experiences, sharing out the goodies, watching the photos and eating. Our return feast was spectacular and every bit as tasty as we had imagined.

After the constant goings on of the last few days, Wednesday and Thursday's pace was totally snail. Sue went home to Biloela and Gav and Al stayed. Andrew pretty much slept the days away, although we gave him a shower late Wednesday afternoon and he quite enjoyed it. The Sleep Centre called and I passed on information about Andrew's condition and improvements he's made. We also had confirmation from one of Andrew's Income Protection claims that the payment had been approved.

On Friday, we made Andrew chicken soup and he had it via the peg. Strangely enough, he tasted it all day and was adamant there was to be no more chicken! We washed Andrew's peg by clamping it off and using hot soapy water and pipe cleaners. As we were giving him food outside of the Fortisip, oil deposits were accumulating on the sides of the tube and needed to be cleared. Gav showed me how to give Andrew one of his antibiotics IV. I don't know who was more afraid — him, Andrew or me — but we all survived.

Saturday 23rd of August; Beau's birthday (my nephew)

Andrew went out to the lounge, although it was under protest. Fan and I had a little trouble manoeuvring him and getting him comfortable and it was quite a testing and frustrating time for all of us. We even had to do some suctioning by ourselves, which was a little daunting given that Fan and I considered ourselves to be assistants-in-nursing-in-training. Poor Andrew. We switched the chicken soup for beef and Andrew stayed out for about five hours before returning to the comfort of his bed.

Following his Sunday morning routine, which included a few bathroom trips, Andrew was quite exhausted and rested for the remainder of the day. He also had some medication to help him settle after the morning's events. He didn't feel up to going out to his chair and we (I) didn't push the issue. We had plans to go to bed early, but then we watched 'The Green Mile' for about the tenth time and it was late when it finished.

Monday wasn't a particularly good day. Sue and Rel tried

Andrew with some porridge and things didn't go well. Andrew couldn't really swallow at all, apart from thin fluids, and while he'd suspected this for a while, actually having it confirmed was very hard to come to terms with. It was difficult to watch and I was really of no help at all as I shed a few tears. We figured we'd put it on the list as one more thing to overcome.

On a more positive note, Rel met with our solicitor re the process of importing the stem cells into Australia. She provided him with information regarding Andrew's condition; a doctor's report and further information about the financial costs would be forwarded once we had it. Dad also picked up the generator and installed it for us. Andrew's mates from the Union were looking after us as the generator was a gift from them.

Andrew's morning routine was extremely drawn out and absolutely exhausting — it lasted around two hours. Needless to say, he was spent for the remainder of the day. We decided to cease the folic acid he was having for the benefit of the stem cells, due to the iron content and the resultant effects it was having on his system.

I escaped to Rockhampton for a few hours and Rel and Fan stayed with Andrew. His Doctor came to visit and was super impressed by Andrew's progress. He said he was happy to share in the miracle — as we all were.

Thursday 28th of August; Rel's birthday

Mum and Dad returned to their 'holiday home' for a few days. I responded to an email from one of Andrew's Union mates regarding the footy match that's scheduled for early November. He was still keen to go out and was more than a little awed that the guys were organising it, but he didn't want to go if he was still on the mask all the time.

As Mum and Dad had gone home, I picked Lainy up from school. When doing so, her teacher mentioned that one of the

Grade One teachers was a Bowen Therapist and the Aide took me to meet with her. After chatting, she indicated a willingness to treat Andrew and she was able to travel to Mount Morgan — wow! Everyone came to our place for dinner for Rel's birthday and she had the night off as Gav and Fan stayed over.

Over the next few days, despite his tiredness, Andrew was not sleeping well, even with the assistance of Midazolam. He was also feeling quite sore in the hip and knee areas. The Sleep Centre called for an update on Andrew's condition and they were going to pass the information we relayed on to the doctors at the Prince Charles Hospital. I went out to Blackwater on Saturday afternoon for a friends Hen's Night, (Rel, Merle and Tay stayed with Andrew), and on my way home Sunday, Rel called to tell me that Andrew was outside in the blue chair! Wow! He was checking out the shed and Gav took him for a stroll around the yard, although it was hard yakka on the grass. Andrew also stayed out in his chair for a while before retiring to the bedroom.

Al was due to come out and stay with us Sunday night, but she didn't as she was ill and didn't want to expose Andrew to anything. Thus, it was just Fan and I. We were a little scared, but we survived. More importantly, so did Andrew! We had a pretty good night and Transformers played on telly so we were happy.

Fan and I did Andrew's morning routine and Gav arrived just as we finished. We were quite proud of ourselves. Our accountant made a home visit to do our tax and true to form, Andrew thought my concept of understanding, or lack thereof, was quite hilarious.

Fan went home Tuesday and Sue returned. Andrew's restlessness continued, but his phlegm was not causing him as much grief. On Wednesday, Andrew showered and sat out in the blue chair for a few hours as some guys came to fix his bed. Strangely enough, the bed couldn't be fixed due to the new cable being faulty. We had the good with the bad though as we were blessed with many visitors — Sam and her new bub, Kelly (Helen's other daughter) and her kids, Fan and Stacey. I sent the faulty BiPAP machine back to Prince Charles Hospital and we had quite a lot of trouble trying to fit Andrew with the Liberty mask. Needless to say, we were all a little cranky by the end of it.

Over the past few days, Andrew felt quite bloated and uncomfortable and as such, he'd not been feeling hungry and this caused some friction as we had been trying to force feed him to ensure he's receiving the necessary nutrients to maintain his wellbeing. The mundane was interrupted by a visit from a friend and as it was Father's Day Night for Lainy's class, we held our own at home. The kids made posters, we had balloons, the kids ate pizza and watched telly in with Andrew and we took some photos of the kids and Andrew for Lainy to take in to school and share. It was actually surprising that Andrew allowed us to take the photos as he was usually more restrained.

Friday 5th of September

Sue stayed home with Andrew while I went to Rocky and visited our rental place at Glendale and did some banking. The day brought more of the same as Andrew had soreness and suffered from phlegm and tiredness. On my return, I talked with Andrew about the morning's events and showed him some pictures of Glendale. Tan and her daughter, Shae also arrived for a visit.

Saturday brought more of the same, but it did herald a new addition. Andrew had his first session of Bowen Therapy as the teacher from Lainy's school visited us. Afterwards, he was ultra-relaxed; as was I as she gave me a treatment as well. It was heavenly.

Sunday 7th of September; Father's Day

The kids were very excited to give Andrew the things they had made for him at school. Andrew was even happy to have his photo taken with the kids. They jumped up in his bed and spent quite a lot of time there throughout the day. We also had quite a few visitors, but as Roy wasn't feeling 100 percent , he had to keep his distance from Andrew.

I wasn't Andrew's favourite person as I wanted him to go out of the room, but he didn't want to. I also wanted to take the computer in and do some things with him, but he wasn't keen. He suffered with chronic wind and while doing his nightly stretches he came out in a rash and was itchy all over. He had to have some Phenergan to settle it.

The following day, Andrew had a shower after the bathroom and it really shattered him. Things were beginning to get really frustrating — for all of us — as it was sometimes difficult to understand Andrew. To make things easier, I brought in Lainy's THRASS chart (language tool) that has sounds/ words and alphabet on it and it seemed to work quite well. We would run our fingers along the chart and Andrew would nod or indicate when we reached the letter/word. We would sometimes even spell things out letter by letter. A basic system, but it worked for us.

As we were travelling to Rocky the next day for Andrew to meet with the Palliative Care Team, we hoped to have an early night. We started Andrew's night routine early, but he still didn't settle and get to sleep until after 1am.

Tuesday 9th of September

We were up early and had finished Andrew's morning routine prior to the ambulance arriving at 8:45am. Rel, Gav and I travelled down with Andrew in the ambulance and the plan was for Andrew to remain on the stretcher during the visit with Palliative Care. On arrival at the hospital, we had to wait to see the doctor and following our meeting with him, we could have waited longer.

We didn't get the impression that he cared overly much about our situation and half way through the consultation, he actually stopped to ask who Andrew was as there were two males! We thought Andrew being on the stretcher and having the BiPAP was a dead give-away, but apparently not. At one point, he said that Palliative Care didn't have a role to play and we should continue as we are. Even when we asked about services he advised that they weren't in a position to provide any as Andrew didn't really fit any of the criteria for them to be involved. Being diagnosed with a terminal illness didn't qualify him for palliative care services — to say we were stunned would be an understatement! I was extremely proud of Rel and Gav for their tremendous self-control and restraint throughout the entire experience. I must note that the interactions we had with other staff at Palliative Care during our visit was very different and more like one would expect it to be.

Andrew's ankles and back were extremely sore and as Gav stayed in Rockhampton, the Ambulance Officers lifted Andrew back into his chair once we were home. It took a little while to get him settled and we gave him some medication to settle.

We discussed putting in a bigger door to the bedroom to allow better access, but Andrew wasn't keen. As it was, if we needed to remove him from the room in a hurry, it would have been very difficult, as only his chair would fit through the opening. Getting him out on his bed would have been impossible and someone suggested taking him out on a blanket and while this sounded quite basic, it would likely have been our best option if the necessity arose.

We started Andrew's routine around 8ish and considering the day he had had, it went really well. He was settled early and amazingly, he was asleep by 11:30pm and he slept soundly for most of the night.

Wednesday was very relaxed compared to the day before. Andrew continued sleeping well and he had a visitor from

Blackwater who updated him on all things happening with the Union. The visit put a spark in Andrew's eye, but hearing of everything that was happening (in our old life) was difficult too, because we are now so far removed from it.

Thursday 11th of September

We visited the Mt Morgan Hospital for a teleconference with Andrew's Brisbane Doctors. Sue left before we did to go to the hospital and when she was leaving, Tank was run over! It was bedlam. Andrew heard it and I saw it. It wasn't Sue's fault as Tank was sleeping under her car (five acres and he chooses to snooze under a car) and due to his deafness, didn't hear it start. If we had any queries about his ability to hear, they were answered by his inaction when the diesel engine rumbled to life and he remained oblivious!

I was a little beside myself, but tried to stay relatively calm as I knew Sue was upset and I didn't want to upset her further by carrying on hysterical. Besides that, it wasn't her fault at all — accidents happen. Luckily, the kids were at school so we didn't have to contend with their reactions straight away. Tank was taken to Rocky and it was a nervous wait until we received the call to say that he needed x-rays and an operation to remove broken teeth. I didn't care what he needed, I just wanted him to be fixed.

Not long after the episode with Tank, we had a visitor who we'd been to school with and hadn't seen in quite a long time. It was a nice distraction, but I must have been a fright as I was still a little freaked out — oh well!

Andrew was transported to the hospital via taxi and it worked out extremely well as he was able to remain in his chair. The video-conference felt a little like our home team versus the opposition, but it was good to share information about how Andrew was going and what had been happening (i.e. our visit to India, the BiPAP machines, Andrew's P.E.G. and our Palliative Care visit). It also allowed us to ask questions about possible procedures that may assist Andrew, such as a tracheotomy. We were just finding out what our options included. Overall, the meeting was better than I had anticipated and it was made all the sweeter as Andrew was able to sit up throughout the entire meeting.

While we had the opportunity, we weighed Andrew whilst at the hospital. He was 97kg, including the chair. Frightening, considering the dramatic difference between now and the beginning of the year.

To say Andrew was tired after the venture out is an understatement of maximum proportion. The events of the last few days and his feeling a little fluey added fuel to the emotional rollercoaster and it was plain exhausting riding the ups and downs. We were also having difficulty in getting thick liquids/ fluids down the P.E.G. due to the wire spring being out of shape in one area and obstructing the flow. Hence, our earlier discussions with the Brisbane doctors, re: a possible replacement.

Andrew didn't have a very good night, as there were issues with the buzzer he used to gain our attention. It wasn't working all the time and this heightened Andrew's and the rest of our anxiety. Rel and Gav fiddled with it and ended up putting a marble on the top, which seemed to work. However, it was all about the hand placement so it wasn't guaranteed.

Due to the increased level of suctioning Andrew required, his throat was quite sore and he had blood blisters in some areas. He also felt unwell/ nauseous and needed some medication to settle. The fact that Tank had to stay another night at the vet may also have been a factor as Andrew was just as worried as I was, if not more because Tank had always been 'his' dog.

Thorlene and I went to Rockhampton on Saturday for a spot of shopping and to pick up Tank. Rel and Gav stayed with Andrew and did his morning routine, which included a shower. One of Andrew's mates called and was going to visit to watch the footy with Andrew as Saint George was playing, but Andrew didn't feel up to the company. His mood worsened when Saint George was beaten and were out of the competition.

Fan and I were on our own from early afternoon. We tried giving Andrew some soup, but it wouldn't go down the P.E.G. so we had to use a suck and plunge technique to clear it. We decided to stick with Fortisip and clear fluids, including the green tea we had been giving him over the last few days.

Andrew had a good night, but he didn't settle until after 1am. We both slept through until around 6:30. Fan woke up a few times during the night and came in and checked on both of us! Rel came out and helped with the morning routine and we had a friend visit after lunch. It was just Fan and I again on Sunday night and while Andrew slept well, he didn't settle until after midnight.

Monday 15th of September

It was quite an emotional day and there were a few tears here and there — frustration, anger, helplessness; pick one! Our entire situation was unreal and when you thought about it, it was more than a little overwhelming. With this, of course, came the feelings of disbelief, hurt, fury, powerlessness and so forth. So, you did the only thing you could do. Somehow you kept going.

Andrew found it hard to get comfortable all day, so we did stretches regularly to alleviate his soreness. We could help Andrew with his external exercises, but those for his breathing and swallowing reflexes were his alone. They certainly weren't easy and sometimes, he found it too difficult to do them at all. We also purchased a pulse oximeter, to help monitor Andrew, especially when he was off the mask.

Fan went home on Tuesday morning and Al came out to stay. Despite having an okay night, Andrew was tremendously tired and wasn't up to his morning routine. He wasn't feeling 100 percent in any sense; he wasn't particularly happy and he didn't want to do anything. We had a visitor from Blackwater after lunch and it seemed to change the atmosphere of the day thus far, as Andrew's sore mood dissipated.

Trueline visited in the afternoon to give a quote on an outdoor area at the back of the house. I discussed things with Andrew, but as he was usually the 'organiser and negotiator' for such things, it must have been particularly frustrating for him to let me have the reins in this instance.

Tuesday night/Wednesday morning was a blur as Andrew was feeling off, very unsettled and uncomfortable and he had little to no sleep. The ill feeling continued throughout the day and while he had medications to counteract it, it didn't really reconcile. Whenever he came off the mask, if only for short periods, he became very red and distressed as a result. His doctor visited and tested Andrew's blood, which showed nothing out of the ordinary. We put in another IV and he had another bag of fluid.

We took Andrew to the bathroom and he had a shower afterwards. In hindsight, the two should have been more spaced out as Andrew was left with no energy or strength.

Thursday proved to be a different day altogether. Andrew went to the bathroom early on with relative ease and the stress was notably less all around. Given his condition of the last few days, we were wondering if he had a slight chest infection and were on the alert re this possibility and taking every precaution possible to ease his predicament.

We had other visitors from Blackwater and to our delight (and horror to the waistlines), we were provided with the most divine array of sweets and yummies. While having visitors from 'home' was comforting in one sense, they were bittersweet in another as it somehow highlighted the chasm between our lives of the present to the past. How quickly things change.

Andrew's feeling generally unwell continued and when we changed his Fentanyl patch on Friday, we realised that he had only had a 12mg patch on since Wednesday. This was less than half of what it should have been as he was used to the 25mg patch. This decrease could have accounted for why Andrew was feeling off over the past few days. A few hours after changing back to the 25mg patch and Andrew was feeling better. It was good to know that his decline of recent days was due to the patch potency and not something more sinister.

Saturday 20th of September

Today heralded Merle and Roy's 50th Wedding Anniversary. Our day progressed as per normal, with lots of umms and ahhs about whether Andrew would come out of the bedroom for the party. I wanted him to come out of the room and join everyone, but he was resistant. It became quite emotional at different times of the day and while Andrew relented and said he would sit out, it never eventuated. Tay did up a slide show for the occasion and as Andrew remained in the bedroom, the 'Unit', Merle and Roy and Stephen (friend, neighbour, brother) all watched it with him ensconced in the room. After the initial showing, everyone had the opportunity to view the show and needless to say, there were plenty of tears free flowing. We also took some photos of everyone together. While we knew that the occasion was special, we didn't realise that these photos would end up being the last ones taken with Andrew and the rest of the family — very special, indeed.

Sunday was a doldrums type of day for the most part, but a visit from some friends soon pepped us up. In its wake, Monday was quite harrowing for lots of reasons. Andrew had quite a traumatic morning with a bathroom visit and shower and his shoulders were extremely sore. His mood was not pleasant and he became quite cranky at times. We were all a little testy and the fact that Andrew's condition seemed to be declining was both a concern and a frustration. Maybe the cells work better when they are administered consistently/on a daily basis as opposed to the quantity of cells? We also emailed our Federal Member (who was in Parliament at the time) regarding our request to have the cells imported.

We also had contact from Brisbane — the M.N.D. nurse and Palliative Care. The latter was 'checking' that Andrew was still the one 'driving the bus' with regard to what was happening with him. Also, on learning of his condition, she indicated that he was at high risk of cardiac arrest due to the stress on his heart when off the mask. Terrifying information, to say the least! Following her contact, we had another 'talk' with Andrew, during which he was very clear in letting us know that he wasn't ready to give up. We fight on. Horrendously emotional chats, but on a positive note, it was good to know everyone was still aiming for the same goal.

Andrew's morning routine and bathroom visit on Tuesday morning were a lot easier than the previous day. We've also been utilising a pulse oximeter (checking the oxygen content in the blood) and his saturation statistics weren't too bad when coming off the mask for short periods. He was having regular doses of Pethidine, which seemed to help him enormously, especially as it allowed him to relax, come off the mask and there was very little redness as a result.

Our day was brightened when we received a reply email from our Federal Member. She had spoken with the Health Minister re Andrew's situation and they were requesting the Form A. Wow! We filled it out, post haste, went and had the doctor sign off on it and faxed it off to the T.G.A.

Wednesday 24th of September

Today saw the Federal Members Office forward a T.G.A. email

to us indicating that the cells would not be allowed into Australia if they were cloned, but there would be no issue if they were harvested. The stem cells are harvested, not cloned, so this was fantastic news, such that we shared our progress with Doctor S. in India. The news also had Andrew quite excited and more animated than he'd been for some time.

Talk about a rollercoaster ride. One day we were down, the next we were up, down, up, down, up. Who needs amusement parks? We were pretty much on the scariest roller coaster ride there ever was.

Andrew had a close friend visit on Thursday and we printed out Doctor S's patent and gave a copy to his doctor as the National Health and Medical Research Council (N.H.M.R.C.) wanted to talk with him about the cells before they made their final decision about importation. Waiting. Waiting. Waiting. In the interim, we carried on as per usual. Andrew's elbows were very sore and we had the ingenious idea of resting them on thawed ice packs to help relieve the pressure and discomfort. It seemed to work okay.

Fan and Rel did a tag on Friday with Fan going and Rel staying. Andrew had another Bowen Therapy session and some reflexology that he found very relaxing. Rel also made contact with the Sleep Centre in relation to Andrew's mouth build-up. Strange as it sounds, we thought he was experiencing a shedding phase and their suggestions were congruent with what we were already practising.

The kids and I went to the beach on Saturday for some down time and Merle and Rel stayed with Andrew. During our absence, Andrew had an episode after having some medication — Maxilon. He came out in a rash and couldn't catch his breath, even on the machine. From all accounts, it was terribly scary. Even more so as he'd had the medication many times previously and had no adverse reaction. He had quite a lot of medication during the day and when doing his nightly routine, he had an enormous amount of phlegm and his throat was very irritated. Rel left after his routine, leaving Al and I on the night shift. Unfortunately, we had to call her back as Andrew required further attention and medication throughout the night. He had phlegm three times during the night and as a result, there was little rest for any of us.

To state the obvious, Andrew didn't have a very good night and he was understandably tired and unsettled during the day. We gave him a shower and tried to make him as comfortable as possible afterwards so he could rest. To our chagrin, Andrew's Liberty mask broke. The clasp snapped while he was wearing it and it was mighty scary, but luckily we had the others on hand and were able to swap them without too much drama. The episode certainly had our blood pumping!

Monday 29th of September

Rel took the faulty mask back and had it exchanged. Andrew needed the mask so we could alternate it with the other, considering there was skin off his nose from the Quattro mask. Aside from some very quick sips of water, each time Andrew comes off the mask, especially during routines, he requires Pethidine . Through trial and error, this medication seems to help him the most and it decreases his distress.

We did Andrew's oral routine three times on Tuesday. It made it a lot easier and cleaner and as much as he didn't like the process, it felt nicer afterwards. Rel had discussions with Palliative Care doctors in Brisbane and they were in support of how we were handling things. They too, were unsure why the Pethidine was having the effect on Andrew that it did and they indicated that the amount he required would likely increase as he built up a tolerance to it, but to continue using it as it worked. Fan and I covered the night shift.

The first of October was heralded by Andrew having another reaction to Maxilon. He was given 5mg initially and all was fine, but on receiving the remainder of the dose, his body reacted. A rash spread over his body and he had the feeling of not being able to catch his breath. It was terrifying to watch his reaction, let alone feel it! Andrew's doctor visited in the afternoon and we advised him of this morning's events. We also had a phone appointment with the Sleep Centre, but as we contacted them when issues arise, there were no outstanding issues.

Rel developed 'elbow doughnuts' out of eggshell mattress as Andrew's elbows were terribly tender and they worked well. In amongst the drama of the day, we freshened Andrew up a little and gave him a shave. He no longer shies away from me with a razor at his throat!

Thursday 2nd of October

Andrew felt off for most of the day and he had recurring heartburn. Strangely enough, and to our delight, he was talking. His voice was very different as it was much deeper and clearer. He asked Sue to move the bed and shift his legs and she was startled to say the very least! We had him saying everything and anything considering he'd not really been talking at all for some time. (It was certainly better than the voice recordings we (I) had been listening to).

Apart from the speech, Andrew had a big day. He went to the bathroom and whilst there, we cut his hair. We're getting quite adept at it too, although it's not Stefan quality and I'm sure they don't vacuum their clients at the time of their style cuts! Not surprisingly, Andrew was quite shattered afterwards and was happy to return to his bed.

We've still not heard any news re importing the cells, but we sent an email to N.H.M.R.C. and followed it up with a phone call. We received an email from our Federal Member on Friday advising we need to approach the N.H.M.R.C. re acquiring a permit to import the cells and all indications thus far regarding this were positive.

Friday also saw Andrew have a longer than usual morning routine as we'd skipped a full one last night due to his fatigue. He was also having trouble with the buzzer again as it wasn't working all the time. We fiddled and tried different things, but there continue to be issues with the system.

Merle is keen to meet with Doctor S. and as she's visiting Australia to attend a Stem Cell Fundraiser, we looked into it. We also had a close friend contact us as she'd heard through the grape vine that Andrew wasn't doing very well. I gave her an update and proceeded to send out an update email.

Saturday 4th of October; Dad's birthday

While Mum and Dad went home to their place, Sue and Rel came to stay at ours. Friends were staying down the beach and they invited the kids and I down to spend the night. It was quite difficult leaving, but it was also nice to get away.

Conflicting emotions are my constant companion. Of course, our friends were curious and concerned and I found that in talking about how things were, I was again struck by Andrew's courage and determination and if it were possible, I was even more proud of him.

The kids and I were home relatively early on Sunday — couldn't stay away for long — and were pleased to find Andrew was doing okay. We did four routines throughout the day and Andrew required around 100mg of Pethidine for each session. He had a very sore thumb on his right hand as it was overextended during a move up the bed. We also ceased pulling him up from under the shoulders as it hurt him too much. We were becoming quite inventive re moving strategies. Despite much thought and ingenuity, there were still buzzer issues, which was an ongoing concern.

The events of early Monday morning will long live in Sue's memory and by mid-morning she had a magnificent bruise on her leg from my Grandma's bed end. Andrew's mask came apart in the middle of the night/morning and Sue was up and doing things before she was even awake! She was on autopilot and despite the leg injury, handled the crisis extremely well. Me, on the other hand, slept through the entire incident! Thank goodness, I wasn't the only one on deck.

As the M.N.D. Association may have been able to assist with resources, especially communication ones (given our dilemma with the buzzer), I contacted them and requested application forms. We also contacted the Australian Quarantine and Inspection Service (A.Q.I.S.) re a permit for the cells as directed by the T.G.A. and N.H.M.R.C. Just our luck though, Canberra were having a Public Holiday and we had to re-contact the following day.

Andrew's electoral forms were also returned to us as I had signed for him as his Power of Attorney. This apparently was not allowed and he needed to sign or make a mark himself — even though he was not able to hold a pen! We could not work this out. I filled out some income protection forms for the month and forwarded them to Andrew's Doctor. Sue returned to Biloela (for a well-deserved break after her extremely stressful couple of days) and Gav came to stay.

Tuesday 7th of October

We made bookings to attend the Stem Cell Fundraiser in Melbourne and contacted the M.N.D. Association to follow up re our request for membership. Andrew went to the bathroom and as it was not a big ordeal, he also had a shower.

M.N.D. Queensland was contacted on Wednesday, re: a different buzzer system, to what we'd been utilizing and we were advised that they would forward what they had. Our system was obviously not working properly and it was a constant source of concern. Andrew was also experiencing mask issues which was very annoying. Gav completed and sent off the permit application to A.Q.I.S. via email and I made Hudson's birthday cake for tomorrow.

For whatever reason, Andrew required larger doses of Pethidine to complete his morning oral routine. He'd also been coughing on and off during the day and on one such occasion, his doctor was present and he listened to Andrew's chest, which was thankfully clear. Around mid-afternoon, Andrew had some Pethidine, which coincided with a coughing fit and wind and we're not sure why, but a rash appeared, Andrew had the sensation of breathlessness and his heart rate accelerated. Even though the machine breathes for Andrew, the sensation of not being able to breathe and his increased heart rate made for a petrifying experience. Rel tried to keep Andrew calm, but the episode lasted quite a while and afterwards, he was totally spent. We were all a little horrified by what happened and as we had Jamie and his wife, Jodie visiting at the time, I told Andrew they'll probably never visit again!

Thursday 9th of October; Hudson's 7th birthday

We had an early start as Hudson opened his presents in our bedroom. This is a family tradition, but this year it was extra special for obvious reasons. I took the kids to Macca's for breakfast and dropped Lainy at school. While Hudson and I were in Rockhampton running errands, Merle and Rel finished off making his birthday cake — it was a chocolate covered piñata.

We tried Andrew with more Pethidine (slower and diluted) to see if he had a reaction. Thankfully, all was fine. We put his previous reaction down to the residual of the drug in his body coupled with wind, coughing and who knows what else! It was just a relief that it was still an option for him. A.Q.I.S. emailed a question in response to our application regarding how the cells would be transported and we answered after contacting Doctor S. re the preferred process.

We had a little party for Hudson in the afternoon and while Andrew stayed in his room, we made videos so he could share in Hudson's day. The fact that no-one could penetrate the chocolate shell of the piñata was cause for more than a few giggles and gaiety, and this frivolity and fun, did not go astray.

Permission Granted

Friday 10th of October

Andrew didn't have a good night as he wasn't able to sleep. He had quite a bit of Pethidine during the night and required more than usual for his morning routine. We had a close friend visit, which was lovely, as despite his tiredness, Andrew was quite animated.

We received correspondence from A.Q.I.S. during the day to say there were no issues with the application for importing the cells thus far. Late in the afternoon, we received spectacular news from A.Q.I.S. — the permit was granted! We were ecstatic, to say the least and emailed Doctor S. straight away. However, amongst the celebration and euphoria, we thought maybe the process was too easy? We weren't used to things being so forthcoming.

While our spirits and hopes were heightened by the days' events, there were others in our lives that had theirs dampened due to personal things they were experiencing. Happiness is a fleeting thing. It should be grasped with both hands while one has the chance to embrace it. Note to self!

Andrew suffered with bad phlegm off and on all of Saturday. We managed through the day, but as it was only Fan and I during the night, we needed to call Gav around midnight to help us as we were unable to administer the medication Andrew required to come off the mask.

Andrew wasn't feeling particularly well on Sunday either and while the plan was for Al to stay, Rel took leave early so she could come out and stay more often. She practically lived at our house when she wasn't at work and sometimes when she was at work anyway. Andrew was quite happy with this course of events as he and Rel were quite the pair — two peas in a pod.

Hudson had a student free day on Monday and he spent quite a bit of time in the room with Andrew. We emailed Doctor S. re where we are at with the import/export of cells. All systems were go on our (Australian) side, but we were not sure where the Indian Government stood.

Tuesday 14th of October

Received correspondence from Doctor S. re she was unable to travel to Australia with the cells, but she had delegated and another doctor would accompany them. Furthermore, from her intel, it could be as soon as next week-end! Things were happening, in addition to the mundane — washing the dogs, organising cabinetmakers for our property at Glendale and doing a quick script run. Despite the great news re the cells and the new buzzer system arriving from the M.N.D. Association, Andrew's condition was not fantastic. He required an enormous amount of Pethidine during his morning routine and while he was up to a shower, the events of the day wore him out totally.

The kids and I went to Rocky on Wednesday to run some errands and while we were away, Sue arrived. Mum and Dad also talked with some friends to procure a caravan for the doctor to stay in whilst they were here. As it was Tank's birthday, we brought him in to see Andrew, which put a smile on his face. It was a bright spot on an otherwise dark day as Andrew wasn't well.

I had to go to Rockhampton again Thursday to do some stuff with our property there. A door was delivered for our patio that was being built and an old friend visited. Andrew was extremely tired and rested most of the day. His eyes were very sore as well. We contacted the M.N.D. Association with regard to an Eye Gaze

System — a computer program that is operated with your eyes — but they were unaware of it. Mum and Dad came up and we did a run through of the generator. I also had a battle with a mouse in the linen cupboard and came out victorious!

Friday 17th of October

Merle, Sue, Fan and I all went to Melbourne to attend the Stem Cell Research Fundraiser and Merle had her wish granted when we met up with Doctor S. It was also a good opportunity to meet with others who have and/or are contemplating having the therapy. We met many people, some of whom had M.N.D. and we shared stories. The majority of people in attendance had spinal injury and while the treatment is the same, it differs in the respect that the cells are targeted at a specific area. With M.N.D., all areas need to be targeted.

Rel stayed with Andrew and during the time we were away, she reported that he wasn't doing well. He was not sleeping, was having difficulty coping with routines and he'd required an enormous amount of medication, just to be comfortable.

Sunday 21st of October

At home, it was almost as if we'd not been away. Not sure about anyone else, but while you're away and doing different activities and such, you're still at home too, because you're constantly wondering what's happening and if all is okay. Home was very busy — Tan and the kids were visiting, Mum and Dad took Lainy to a birthday party before bringing the kids home and we had one of Andrew's Union mates visit. Our shed was finished and arrangements made for the concrete to be poured for the patio.

Whilst all this was going on, Andrew's condition was very poor. He was unable to withstand any form of his morning or nightly routine, couldn't breathe, had sore eyes and felt exhausted.

The D.O.N. visited and confirmed Andrew's critical status. We tried to make him as comfortable as possible, with company, care and medications.

Further enquiries were made with regard to the Eye Gaze System on Monday and information was requested. Calls were also made regarding the mounting of our bedroom air conditioner converter, as it needed to be done in order for the patio to proceed.

Contact was made with the N.H.M.R.C. and the T.G.A. in relation to the cell importation. We were still waiting on word from the Indian Government re where they stood on the issue. It was becoming increasingly clear that Andrew's condition was not improving and his need for the cells was immediate. While in India and receiving the treatment regularly, signs of improvement were evident, but the decline in his condition had been obvious since the cell treatment had ceased.

Considering Andrew's dire need of cells, we contacted Doctor S. on Tuesday to get an update on the Indian side of things. She'd not had any further correspondence from said Government, but would advise once she had. We also contacted our solicitor to clarify the process. He did some homework and re-contacted with information regarding jurisdiction, deeds of indemnity, terms of agreements between parties and so forth. It certainly was a conundrum.

We had a close friend call to see how Andrew was travelling. All things considered, he was doing okay. However, there had been little positive change in his condition for some time and as much as it rallied us when his condition improved, such improvements weren't maintained. As bystanders, we were again on a roller-coaster ride. Sadly, however, Andrew was the track as he was being twisted and turned and one must think, found it very difficult to keep the mechanics of everything going.

Wednesday 22nd of October

Friends of Mum and Dad dropped off a caravan in anticipation of the Indian Doctor's visit. We thought they would be more comfortable in their own accommodations as opposed to staying in the house with us. We also had contact with Doctor S. regarding how the cells would be transported so we would be ready and organised once given the final approval. Following this contact, we surfed the net, searching for appropriate freezers and transport companies.

Andrew was very tired and the buzzer was still causing havoc. As such, if someone was not in the room with him all the time, we would check on him in very regular intervals. One positive though, we were trialing a film of Vaseline in Andrew's mouth, in an effort to prevent build up and to keep his mouth moist, and it appeared to be working quite well. Anything positive was welcomed, no matter how small or significant it may or may not be.

Concrete for the back patio was poured on Thursday and the materials for the construction itself were delivered. I did a school run to Rockhampton to pick up Lainy and we called ahead and collected some scripts for Andrew as well.

All was not good, however, as Merle was unwell. She was taken to hospital, saw the doctor and underwent various tests. It was really no surprise to find that her condition was caused by stress!

Andrew was also having another 'off' day. He felt as though he couldn't catch his breath, which was likely related to his severe wind. He also felt nauseous and as such, didn't have his nightly oral routine. We did, however, do his physical stretches and such, even though they were sometimes uncomfortable and painful.

Throughout Thursday night/Friday morning, Andrew was very restless and didn't get a lot of sleep. He had constant pain and soreness and required medication to ease it and help him settle.

'OOO' Week

Friday 24th of October

The day started off as any other with our doing a short morning routine, which was hampered by Andrew's tiredness. Calls were also made re the Eye Gaze System, patio concrete, which had lots of cracks and an order was put in for a door for the patio.

In the early afternoon, Rel, Merle, Andrew and I were the only ones at home. I had been putting clothes on the line and had heard Andrew's buzzer go off. As Rel had gone in for a shower, I was going back to our room, but when I passed the bathroom, I heard a sickening thud and following that, primal grunts and other horrifying sounds. I tried the door, but it was locked.

TERROR! I tried to remain calm, considering Merle's episode yesterday, I didn't want to alarm her any more than necessary and on my way out to get a knife to unlock the door, I saw Andrew looking at me from our room and he looked as terrified as I felt. I told him what I was doing and while getting the knife, I asked Merle to come in with me as I thought Rel had hurt herself in the bathroom.

To our horror, we found Rel on the floor and it was obvious that she had fallen and hit her head as she was still on the floor, there was blood everywhere and she wasn't conscious. Merle sat with her, I went and told Andrew what was happening to try and alleviate some of his distress and then I contacted '000'. I also called Gav and he wasted no time in getting to us. He beat the ambulance!

By the time the ambulance arrived, Rel was conscious and moving around, but she was not at all well. We tried to settle her, but she was determined to get to Andrew and nobody was going to stop her. Once she was in with Andrew, her presence both reassured and horrified him. Funnily enough, her being in with Andrew seemed to calm her somewhat and things progressed to the point whereby she was amenable to being taken out to the ambulance and subsequently, to the hospital.

Rel was taken to Rockhampton for a CT scan, which was thankfully clear, but she had to stay overnight in hospital. Gav stayed with Andrew, Sue and Fan came up and I went to Rockhampton to pick up Lainy and check in on Rel.

Needless to say, Rel's accident had a titanic effect on everyone, but none more so than Andrew. I'll never forget the look in his eye's; being able to hear and to some extent, see what was going on, but being powerless to stop it or do anything to change it. It's one thing to not be able to help himself, but something different altogether that he's not able to help someone else. It's a look I wish never to see again in anyone's eyes.

The mood that afternoon was quite sedate and all the excitement, albeit not good, had us all quite upset. We did Andrew's nightly routine and due to lots of different factors, it took eons, around three hours to complete and quite a lot of medication. None of us rested well that night.

In the wake of yesterday, Saturday was quite reserved. Andrew was quite out of sorts, but then, we all were. His morning routine went well compared to that of last night and we gave him a shave. His elbows continued to give him grief so we did what we could.

We sent Doctor S. an email on 'cryoport' re a transportation method for the cells for her input and we had quite a few phone calls throughout the day, some wanting progress reports on Andrew, others wanting them on Rel, who was let out of hospital and went home. The kids were due to sleep at Merle's, but Lainy ended up coming home.

Sunday 26th of October

The concrete on the back patio had been broomed off as a result of the cracking and while we weren't 100 percent satisfied, it was certainly better than how it was. I imagine it made Andrew more than frustrated not being able to take control of the situation, as he would have done before becoming ill.

The Pethidine chart we were using appeared to be working well and aside from its other applications, this particular medication appeared to dry up Andrew's phlegm, thus decreasing the amount of suction he required.

While Rel visited, she didn't help out with Andrew's routine and shower and after a while, she became unwell and went home. This wasn't to be the last of the drama, however, as Merle decided to take the spotlight.

There was a game of some description going on at the table when Merle started to feel poorly and next minute, she had collapsed and was on the floor! While she was being tended to, I called '000' for the second time in three days. Unbelievable as I'd never called it ever before!

Even though the service had only been out to our place a few days before, to our disbelief, the ambulance went to the wrong house! We sent Jordan (Al's son) down to the corner on a push-bike to tell them where we were. It came out that our address/road is not on the ambulance/emergency system, which is of grave concern. Merle was taken to hospital and kept in overnight for observation.

Monday was quite busy as calls were made to Doctor S. re the cell transportation, the T.G.A. re Doctors' letters, the Rockhampton Grammar School re Hudson having a confirmed place for next year and '000' re our not being on their system. Regarding the latter, we stressed the importance of their knowing where we are, given our circumstances. Information was also sent to friends in Blackwater, relating to Andrew, for the upcoming football match — B.M.A. Panda's Bears versus Curragh Miners.

Merle was taken to Rocky for further tests and much to her disgust, stayed another night in hospital. Andrew didn't really have a good day as he had difficulty sleeping, was very tired, had sore elbows, phlegm, mask problems and pain. Both Sue and I stayed in with Andrew and as was the norm, the TV went non-stop. Ironically, Andrew enjoyed watching cooking shows — quite cruel really as he couldn't taste/experience any of the wares. He also enjoyed watching Australian Idol and it became a bit of a custom for all of us to pile into our room and watch it together. Funnily enough, when we were in Blackwater and Australian Idol came on, I'd have to go and watch it in the bedroom!

On Tuesday, we had further correspondence with friends in Blackwater regarding the footy game they were pulling together for Andrew. While we all hoped for Andrew to attend, it was very much a wait-and-see until closer to the time, especially considering the two-hour drive and Andrew's comfort level. Seemed silly, putting so much thought into his travelling a few hours when you consider he'd been to India twice. However, his condition was not the same as it was and this needed to be taken into consideration.

We were contacted by another family who was experiencing similar challenges to us as one of their loved ones had M.N.D. On top of this, we received a call from Palliative Care in Brisbane.

Merle was released from hospital and visited and Helen was put in hospital in Rockhampton overnight for an unrelated procedure. What is it with the Curtis clan and hospitals?

Doctor S. called with news that she was expecting to hear back from the Indian Government in the next two to three days. In the meantime, she was trying to arrange a Visa for the accompanying doctor and she requested we send a letter of invitation to said doctor in support of her application.

Andrew's soreness and pain continued, as did his inability to sleep. Even with Midazolam, he was only having short sleeps. Despite this, his routines were bearable.

The invitational letter to the Indian Doctor was sent on Tuesday and wonders would never cease, I actually planted some plants. Everyone knows I am so not a green thumb!

Andrew's doctor visited and reiterated his support of what we were doing and his being behind us all the way. He also had contact from Palliative Care in Brisbane and together we were trying different combinations of medications to make Andrew as comfortable as possible. He was not doing fantastically well as he was always tired and not having sound sleep. Even with medication, he was only sleeping two to three hours at a time, which was proving to be a detrimental pattern. He also had sore eyes, elbows and the masks were proving difficult.

Thursday 30th of October

Contacted Suncorp about an insurance issue at our Glendale property, put in another script for Andrew, called re the Eye Gaze System, hunted down and made purchases off the ice-cream man and received calls from friends. Helen also came out and her daughter, Sam, visited. One would think it was just another day. It wasn't.

While we were doing Andrew's morning routine, a combination of things caused him to pass out. It was very scary. While Rel and Sue stayed with him and did what they do, I contacted '000' for the third time in a week! Rel was shouting out information for me to pass on to the ambulance, which was a little confusing until I relayed our circumstances. The ambulance arrived, provided the necessary medications and Rel administered them. The D.O.N. also came out and we were all extremely relieved when Andrew opened his eyes. Given our situation, it was decided that

Andrew wouldn't be transported to the hospital for follow-up as we could do it at home.

In the aftermath, we were all on the other side of weary and Sue had hurt her back in all the commotion. As a result, Gav came to help out with the nightly routine.

As the kids were at school when everything happened, I let them know later that we had to call an ambulance for their dad and gave them a brief overview of the events. Knowing what to tell them and what to keep from them was not always an easy choice, but one thing remained the same, we didn't hide anything from them. Some details were omitted here and there and things explained in a simpler context, but the crux of all that was happening was laid out for them. In scenarios where the future is unwritten, we thought it unwise to foster false hope or protect the kids from what was really happening — painful, but necessary.

Sue's back was ridiculously sore on Friday and she needed medication to ease the pain and was laid up next to Andrew. Also in relation to medication, had discussions with Palliative Care in Brisbane re Andrew's episode yesterday and the role that medications may or may not, have played in it. Furthermore, discussions were had on how to proceed here-on-in.

During Andrew's routines, he indicated that he was having the same feelings as yesterday and we thought something must have been triggering a like-response during his mouth care. Luckily, yesterday's events weren't repeated, but at the end of the day, Andrew was really, really tired.

Over the week-end, the kids and I went toy shopping, Mum, Dad, Tan and the kids, some close friends and my Aunty Tricia came to visit, I stalked and bettered a mouse in the pantry and a letter was sent to the Australian Consulate in India regarding the Indian doctor visiting us and bringing the cells. Rel wasn't faring well, but she stayed on regardless and when Fan went home on Sunday, Sue and I continued on.

We started Andrew back on everything in preparation for his receiving the cells. We were all a little emotional and it was apparent that Andrew was finding it difficult to cope with reduced amounts of some medications. Additionally, he had a sore nose from the masks and there was blood in the back of his throat from the constant use of the sucker.

The information pertaining to the Eye Gaze System finally arrived on Monday. On reading it, it seemed to be just what we were looking for to make things easier for Andrew to communicate with us. We ordered a demonstration and following that, we could arrange a trial of the system, which we were all excited about.

Lainy had a couple of really severe nosebleeds during the day and she caught the bus home from school in the afternoon. We made contact with Customs and sent Doctor S. an email regarding the cells and while Gav had helped Al and I with the morning and nightly routines, it was just Al and I through the night.

Tuesday 4th of November; Melbourne Cup Day

Trueline were proving difficult as they were due to arrive and start work on the patio yesterday, but were still to present themselves. Notwithstanding this or anything else that was going on, we were true to the season and held a luncheon, complete with dress ups and hats. Andrew was the judge of fashions in the field and we all had an okay time, considering. Al stayed again and despite Andrew's shoulders being really sore and wind making him nauseated, the night passed without too much drama.

We'd had contact from Doctor S.'s associate regarding approval for the mode of cell transportation so Rel was onto it on Wednesday, contacting the various transport companies and refining details. We advised Doctor S. of our progress and we also received a letter from the N.H.M.R.C.

Lainy had a doctor's appointment and she had bloods taken, just to be on the safe side. When she was three, she had Transient Erythroblast of Childhood, which required her to have a blood transfusion. Thus, anything to do with her and blood (i.e. nose-bleeds or paleness), we were a little paranoid. She was quite happy though, given she had the day off school.

One of Andrew's Union mates visited and we discussed things associated with Andrew's employment and sadly, we nominated a date of termination from his position. While this was inevitable, actually making it a reality was very confronting and it stirred up quite a lot of emotion.

Andrew's shoulders continued to bother him so we brought a brace for him to wear to support them. We also decided he needed a more supportive pillow for his neck as it lolls to the right.

Thursday didn't start off very well as the fellow from Trueline arrived to start erecting the patio, but due to the fixings thus far, he refused to put it up! With clenched teeth, we made arrangements for a meeting of the parties involved to occur on Tuesday. I'm sure if Andrew was able, he would have had a few things to say! As it was, I got the gist of what he would say just with a glance.

Mum, Dad and Sue all went home, I picked up the girls in Rockhampton, ran some errands and on returning home, Andrew and I looked up cars and things on the laptop. He'd been doing okay, but that could have been attributed to the fact he'd had more Pethidine than usual, given his constant pain.

Gav had to come out and stay on Friday as Rel had to go to the hospital. She had an arm infection that originated from the contrast they injected when doing tests following her head injury two weeks ago! Despite this, she came back out after leaving the hospital. Fan was due to come up, but she was sick and decided to stay home. Tan and the kids arrived for a visit and Lainy's blood tests all came back negative, which was a relief.

Not much seemed to get past Andrew and during the night, he kept buzzing to make sure that Rel was taking her medication!

Saturday 8th of November; Panda's Footy Match

Unfortunately, Andrew was in no condition to make the trip out to Blackwater for the Footy Match. Gav, Rel and Fan stayed with him and quite a few of us attended on his behalf. The whole weekend was quite surreal. Just returning to Blackwater was a bit of an emotional ordeal as it was the first time the kids and I had been back since leaving. Prior to the event even starting, we were catching up with friends and it was all a little overwhelming.

Nothing, however, compared to what it was like arriving at the football grounds. The sky was ominous and there were severe weather warnings, but regardless, the grounds kept filling up. There was a constant stream of people and it was literally standing room only. The crowd was unbelievable and to think that they had all come out in support of Andrew was insane, staggering and extremely touching. I tried to keep Andrew and the others at home updated, but it was difficult to convey all that was happening.

The actual football game itself was amazing and each player undoubtedly put their heart and soul into the game. The teams were ferocious and I actually felt privileged to watch it. The passion and commitment shown by the players was a credit to them and it was entirely humbling.

The night seemed to have it all. The battle on the field was only marginally seconded by the electrical storm and downpour that occurred part way through the game and while both teams deserved to win, Panda's Bears came away with the victory. It was a very proud moment when Hudson presented the Captain of Panda's Bears with the trophy. It was very fitting too, as the Captain was a close friend and instrumental in the night's conception and it coming to fruition.

Following the game, there was an auction and the tremendous support continued. Everything from the people who played in the game, made donations, purchases, helped out with the game, serving behind the counters — it was all appreciated more than they knew.

I was more than a touch nervous as I gave a little speech, but in the circumstances, it was the least I could do. By the same token, I felt it was totally inadequate considering what the people of Blackwater, our hometown, were giving us in return. Knowing that you are not alone and you have the support of others is sometimes worth more than anything else.

On our return to the Mount, we had a wealth of tales to tell of last nights' events and while Andrew was soaking up the stories, they were somewhat bittersweet as he was unable to experience them himself and I'm sure our recollections didn't do the event justice.

Tan and the kids left early as she was feeling a little unwell and didn't want to share whatever it was she had. The D.O.N. came out with Andrew's medications and alterations were being made to his medication regime to suit his ever-changing condition. As such, the monitoring of his condition and his response to the medications was paramount. Andrew was also a veritable gauge, as he could indicate when he wasn't feeling 'right'.

Following the events of the weekend, Hudson and Lainy took their special 'Panda's Bears' jerseys to school on Monday, for Show and Tell. One of Andrew's close mates called and sent some photos through of the Footy Match, which were very well received. I also sat with Andrew and penned a 'Thank You' letter to be published in the Blackwater paper. We were both a little teary by the end of it.

Rel still had trouble with her arm and had to go to Rockhampton for an ultrasound. It showed that she had an abscess and it needed to be surgically drained. Despite this, she returned to our place and her, Fan and I did Andrew's routine. Andrew's quite sore all over, especially his back and although the skin wasn't broken, we put some extra padding on to try and make him more comfortable.

Running Out of Time

Tuesday 11th of November

We had a very early and terrifying start to the day. Around 5am, Andrew had an episode whereby he couldn't breathe and was freaking out. He spelt out, 'This is it', on the chart and following that, he spelt, 'kids'. He settled after having some medications, but he asked to be 'knocked out' as he couldn't stand the feeling of not being able to breathe and he had a tightness in his chest and back.

I wasn't in the best of places, given the morning's events, but I tried to carry on. I kept the kids home from school and everyone came out throughout the day. Even though Andrew was out of it for most of the day, his room was never empty as we were all in and out. The morning's episode was a reality check.

The kids had an activity day at Rel's on Sunday, thanks to Tay and her school buddies. Sue went home and we had contact from Dr S. saying there was still no word from the Indian Government. As there had been no precedent, no-one really knew how to proceed, so it appeared the process had stalled.

During Andrew's nightly routine, his airway became blocked and he choked. It was very, very scary. We were all on high alert afterwards, but the remainder of the routine was free of any further crisis. The night was not without them, however, as in the early hours of the morning, Rel's 'weird feeling' returned as she was having a reaction to the medications she was on for her arm!

There were lots of forms to be filled out on Monday relating to Andrew's various TPD's, his new RESMED machine arrived and we continued working on Hudson's school project. We also had to deal with Andrew having another episode, whereby he became totally unresponsive, his heart rate plummeted dramatically and he needed emergency medications to rouse him. His doctor and the D.O.N. came out afterwards and while their presence intensified the severity of the situation, nothing, but the look in Andrew's eyes, could have made it more obvious that things were very much hanging in the balance.

You wouldn't credit it, but in the middle of the episode, a representative from the High Commission of India rang to discuss our application for the importation of cells and none of us were available to talk with them because of everything else that was going on!

It all seemed to be playing out like a stage show and you were kept on the edge of your seat because you didn't know what was going to happen next. The show was most definitely a dramatic thriller and while you yearned to leave the theatre, you couldn't leave your seat.

Tuesday 18th of November; our 8th Wedding Anniversary

The fact that it was our anniversary made the day special and given its significance, I was more prone to whimsy and melancholy. Andrew had had a really bad night and his breathing issues continued, so the last thing I was expecting was for him to remember or even acknowledge our anniversary, let alone conspire with others to make something of it.

Regardless of how or why, we had not had an anniversary where Andrew hadn't brought me roses. You can't imagine my surprise when I went in to our room and there was a bunch of twelve red roses sitting on Andrew's lap and he was just giving me that look. I folded like a wet tissue and had a little (or rather large) emotional moment. It was a treasured moment.

I found out later that he had somehow asked his Mum to get me the roses and she and my Mum had told me porky pies about where they were going and why to cover up what they were really doing. I was totally clueless, which is not that much of a surprise. Merle also found a heart-shaped balloon that said, 'Today, Tomorrow and Forever. I love you.' The sentiment was not lost on either of us.

Our thank you letter to all involved in the Footy Match was printed in the Blackwater Herald and I penned a letter on Andrew's behalf to the Union, thanking them for all their support.

A representative from the High Commission of India called back and requested all of our documentation. Preliminary indications were that our application would be approved for the importation of stem cells into Australia. While we were ecstatic re this news, the time factor was seemingly overriding, given Andrew's condition.

Andrew's oxygen saturation levels had been quite low, he'd had a lot of medications and was barely maintaining a comfortable level, he was refusing to do his routines and was having difficulty keeping his mouth open when we did do them. He also indicated that he preferred sedation to the constant struggle.

Wednesday didn't bring any peace. Andrew was very emotional early on, revealing that he felt that his condition was getting worse and the cells had a 'big' job to do, when or if they ever got here. The D.O.N. visited again and did a blood gas test, the results of which were not favourable. There was also talk of his having infusions of certain medicines to ease his pain and discomfort.

We had quite a few friends call and ask if they could visit, but Andrew wasn't up to having visitors. He was having difficulty concentrating and staying in the moment with us.

We also received notice that our insurance claim for Glendale had been approved, I washed our mobile phone, had a Sleep

Centre appointment and dealt with the ongoing dramas of Trueline and the patio.

Andrew's condition didn't really improve overnight and on Thursday, he was having regular doses of medication to keep him settled. He was also having oxygen and Ventolin in an effort to make him feel better. He had the breathless sensation all day and didn't want to do anything, not even change masks. The D.O.N. came out to see how he was travelling.

That night, I talked with Hudson again about his dad being very sick. It was a very difficult conversation and he had a lot of questions that I couldn't answer. It broke my heart.

Friday 21st November; Sue's birthday; Andrew's Star Day

Andrew didn't have a good night and the morning heralded no improvement. He was very emotional and despondent; asking how long he had. A week? A year? Rel also told me of Andrew's response when Hudson went in the room to talk with him before school. Her description of the pain, anguish and struggle she saw in Andrew's eyes as he tried to engage with Hudson and stay with him in that moment was heartbreaking. Once Hudson left the room, Rel said Andrew just looked at her, and she knew.

At one point through the morning, Andrew had me get the computer as he wanted to go through information pertaining to our real estate and some other things he thought important we revisit. I remember us having a battle of wills as I didn't see the need or believe he was up to the task, given how he'd been feeling. Little did I know, or want to acknowledge at the time. Essentially, I imagine he was wanting to tie up loose ends, so I wouldn't have to. He was always thinking of me.

Rel, Gav and I talked about Andrew and what we could do, knowing that he would never give up the fight — he would never give up on us. We talked about his fighting spirit, but we also faced the reality of his weakened body and its inability to keep going. We talked about how hard it must be for him, being in that position of constant fear and not having any control. We talked about being fair to him and what would be best for him and in doing so, decided that we would do for him what he couldn't do for himself.

We all stuck close during the remainder of the day and on leaving to go and get Hudson from school, I ducked in to our bedroom and said, "I'll be back soon Darl, I'm just going to pick up Hudson." These would be the last words I would say to Andrew. When we returned home, he was sedated. Rel said that as soon as I was gone, Andrew indicated that he wanted to do his routine, despite the fact that he'd been avoiding it for the past two days as each time it was more difficult and he was continually passing out. In a way, I guess it was his way of taking control and I believe that he was protecting me to the very end. He always liked to have the last word.

We contacted everyone and they all came. We also invited the D.O.N. to be with us, because we knew that none of us could complete the deed that would give Andrew the ultimate release.

I took Lainy and Hudson into our room and we sat with Andrew. He looked so peaceful. The kids talked to him, told him they loved him and they each gave him a kiss.

Over the course of the afternoon, people went in and had their time with Andrew and once everyone had arrived, Mum and Dad had the children outside and...

Our room was full of people, but as we savoured your presence, we each could have been alone with you in an empty space. The atmosphere was palpable and the mood sombre, but most of us were oblivious to our surroundings as our individual memories, hopes, thoughts and emotions took precedence.

Just as we knew that you would never give up, we also knew that you could no longer go on. With much deliberation, this premise, along with a fathomless well of love, saw your mask removed for the very last time. After having tried so hard for so long to keep your mask on and knowing what its absence personified, seeing you without it was quite surreal and painful beyond words.

In that moment, you were both set free and condemned.

As you lay before me, I looked at you without the mask that had somehow become a part of you and I saw the man that you had always been — my partner in life and love, the father of my children and my hero. Acute sadness engulfed me as images of what should have been our future flashed before me — celebrating birthdays, anniversaries, attending graduations, teaching Hudson to shave, driving lessons, buying Hudson his first car, walking Lainy down the aisle at her wedding and just growing old and being together.

At the same time, I was thankful for the life that we had shared and the many joys that we had experienced together. I was grateful that we had found one another so early on in our lives and the knowledge that what we had shared was very precious and rare was of great comfort. I was also overwhelmed with love and pride and I was in awe of your supreme strength of will, determination and non-defeatist attitude.

As I held your hand in mine and rested my other hand over your heart, time was suspended. You looked so peaceful; as though you were sleeping. But you weren't sleeping. With every beat of your heart and with every tear that fell, your life force was ebbing away.

Baboom… Baboom... Baboom... Baboom... and then you were gone.

Friday, 21st of November 2008, 7pm.

New Releases... also from Sid Harta Publishers

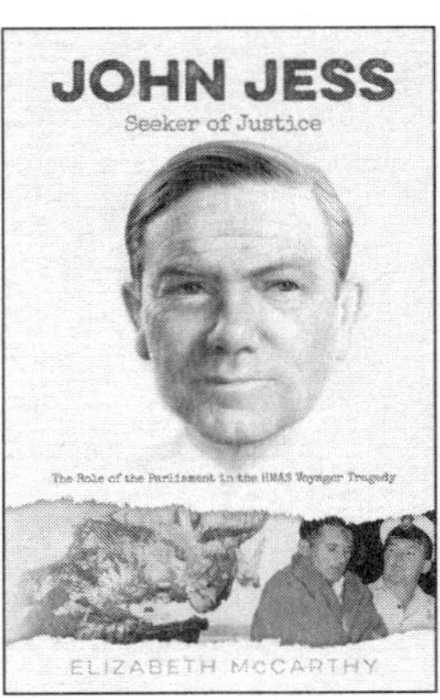

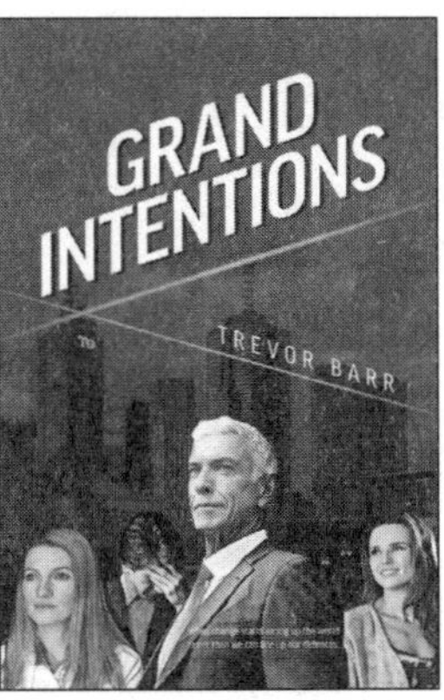

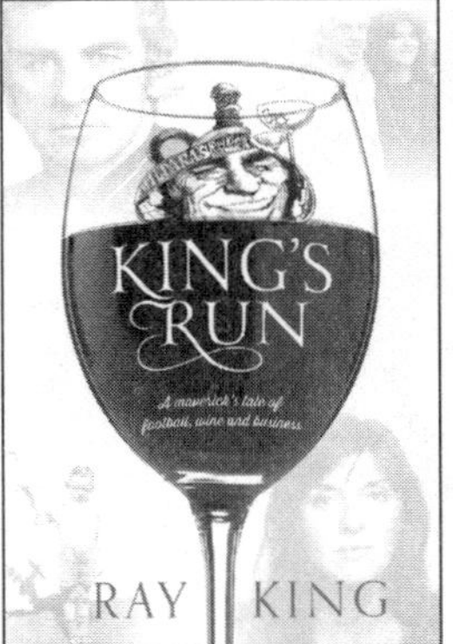

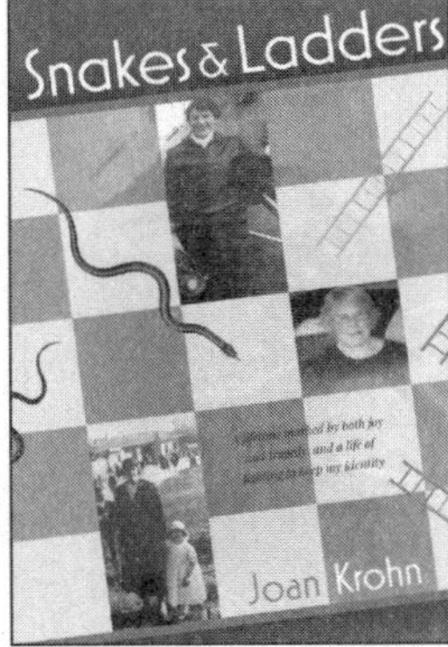

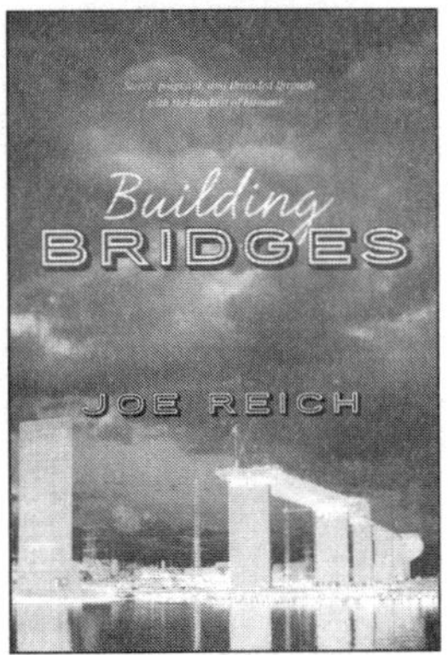

Best-selling titles by Kerry B. Collison

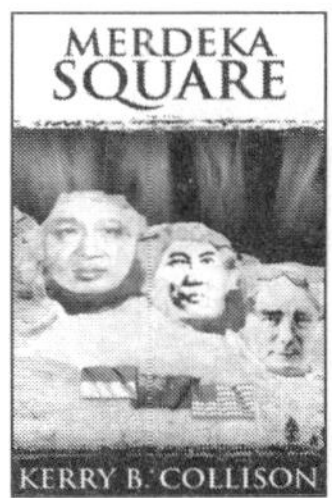

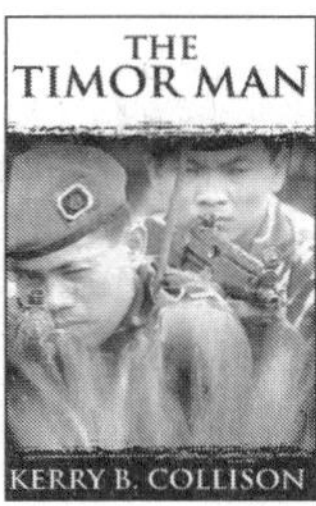

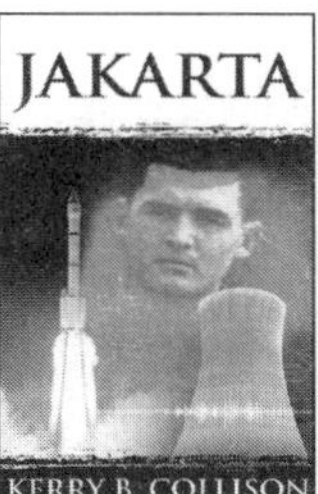

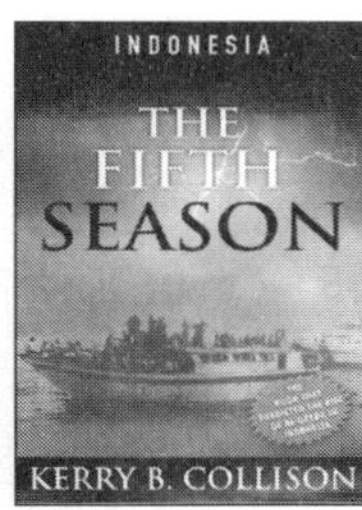

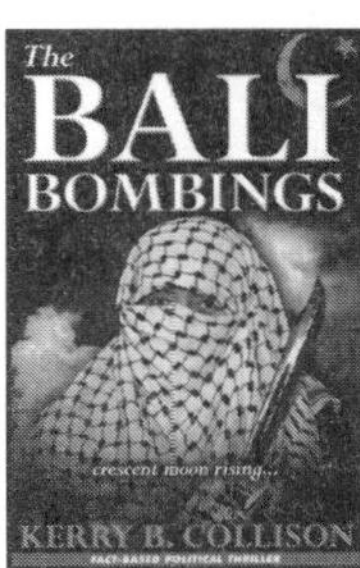

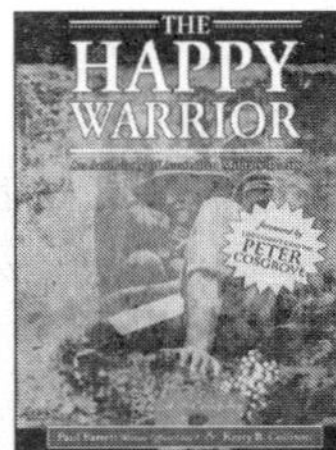

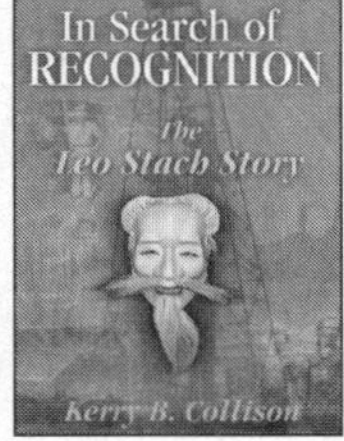

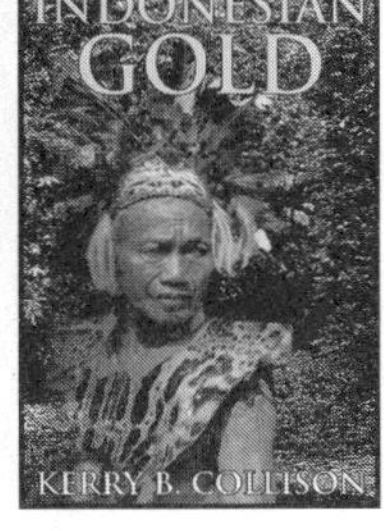

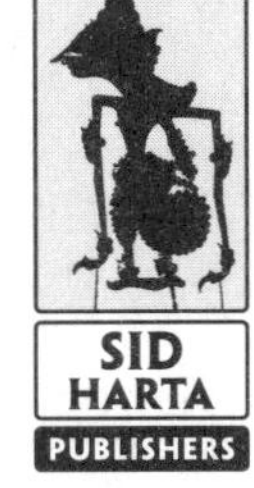

Readers are invited to visit our publishing websites at:
http://sidharta.com.au
http://publisher-guidelines.com/
Kerry B. Collison's home pages:
http://www.authorsden.com/visit/author.asp?AuthorID=2239
http://www.expat.or.id/sponsors/collison.html
email: author@sidharta.com.au

Purchase Sid Harta titles online at:
http://sidharta.com.au